DASH DIE

PROTECT YOUR HEART

A Heart Healthy Cookbook With Effective Recipes To Fight High Blood Pressure and Lower Cholesterol - Meal Prep Cookbook

VINCENT INGRAM

from the Publisher. All additional right reserved.

The information in the following pages is broadly considered to be a truthful and accurate account of facts and as such any inattention, use or misuse of the information in question by the reader will render any resulting actions solely under their purview. There are no scenarios in which the publisher or the original author of this work can be in any fashion deemed liable for any hardship or damages that may befall them after undertaking information described herein.

Additionally, the information in the following pages is intended only for informational purposes and should thus be thought of as universal. As befitting its nature, it is presented without assurance regarding its prolonged validity or interim quality. Trademarks that are mentioned are done without written consent and can in no way be considered an endorsement from the trademark holder.

Table of Contents

PART I

Chapter 1: Introduction to the Heart-Healthy Diet

A heart-healthy diet is incredibly important. The truth is, you must be able to manage your diet well if you want to be healthy. The average diet is actually incredibly unhealthy for the heart, and the sooner that you are able to change up how you treat yourself and your body, the better off you will be. The average person consumes far too much salt and not enough of the important fruits and veggies that they need. As a result, they wind up with problems with their blood sugars, their blood pressure, and cholesterol levels. It is important to understand that your heart is one of the most important parts of your body—you cannot live without it. You need to keep it healthy. If you want to ensure that you can keep yourself healthy, you need to make sure that you eat the foods that will help you to nourish it readily. The sooner that you can do so, the better off you will be. This book is here to provide you with plenty of heart-healthy meals that you can enjoy that will help you to stay as healthy as possible.

The Rules of the Heart-Healthy Diet

Before we begin, let's go over some of the most important rules that go into the heart-healthy diet. These are rules that will help you to ensure that your body is kept as healthy as possible with foods that will nourish you well. Now, on this diet, you can expect to follow these rules:

1. **Decrease saturated and trans fats:** These are fats that are no good for anyone. Instead, it is recommended that you focus entirely on monounsaturated and polyunsaturated fats. These come from primarily vegetarian options—common sources include olive and canola oils, avocado, nuts, and fatty fish.

2. **Increase fruits and veggies:** Your body needs the vitamins and minerals in fruits and veggies to stay as healthy as possible. You should be consuming at least seven to nine servings per day to keep your body healthy and on track.

3. **Consume more fiber:** Typically, on this diet, you want to up your fiber intake. Fiber is necessary to keep your body regular. It also helps

with the way that you will naturally digest and absorb nutrients. You need both soluble and insoluble sources to stay as healthy as possible. Soluble fiber will aid in regulating your body and is fantastic for the heart. Insoluble fiber is there to help you regulate your weight and pass waste.

4. **Make the switch to plant proteins whenever possible:** You will also see that this diet advocates for more vegetarian options and less meat. While you can still eat meat, it is highly recommended that you choose to put in at least three servings of vegetable proteins, and you limit red meats down to just once a week. Twice a week, you should eat skinless poultry, and twice a week, you should enjoy fish.

5. **Up your whole grain intake:** This is essential to ensuring that you are not just consuming a bunch of empty carbs that aren't doing anything for you. By shifting to whole grains, you get more of the fiber that you need, and they are also usually full of better nutritional content as well.

6. **Limiting sweets:** If you are going to enjoy sweets, it is usually recommended that you cut out sugar or sugar-sweetened dishes. While you do not have to completely eliminate them, you should, at the very least, monitor and regulate intake.

7. **Low-fat dairy products:** You should have between two and three servings of dairy per day, but they ought to be reduced fat.

8. **Drink in moderation:** Alcohol is okay—but is not really encouraged either. If you must drink alcohol, make sure that you do so in moderation, which is typically defined as no more than one per day for women and no more than two per day for men.

The Benefits of the Heart-Healthy Diet

The heart-healthy diet has all sorts of benefits that are worth enjoying, and you should be able to treat these as motivation. If you find that you are struggling to enjoy this diet, consider these benefits to give you that added boost. Ultimately, the heart is the key to the body, and if you can keep it healthier, you will enjoy a better life for reasons such as:

- **Preventing heart disease:** When you limit salts, sweets, red meats, and everything else, you will help your heart remain healthier, and in doing so, you will reduce your risk of both stroke and heart disease.

- **Keeping your body healthier:** This diet is often recommended to older people, and this is for good reason—it keeps the body more agile by reducing the risk of frailty and muscle weakness.

- **Cutting the risk of Alzheimer's disease:** This diet helps your cholesterol, blood sugar, and blood vessel health, all of which are believed to aid in reducing the risk of both dementia and Alzheimer's disease.

- **Cutting the risk of Parkinson's disease:** Similarly, because this diet will be high in antioxidants, it has been found to cut the risk of Parkinson's disease significantly.

- **Longer lifespan:** This diet, because it lowers your risk of heart disease and cancer, is actually able to reduce your risk of death by around 20%.

- **Healthier mind:** If you suffer from anxiety or depression, this diet can actually help to alleviate some of the symptoms, or keep them at bay in the future. Between the healthy fats, rich vegetable content, and the boost to your gut bacteria, you will find that your body and mind both are healthier than ever.

- **It helps manage weight:** If you have struggled with your weight for some time, you may find that using this diet will actually help you to manage it, thanks to the fact that you'll be cutting out much of the foods that tend to lead to weight gain in the first place. You'll be able to enjoy a healthier body as the weight fades away through enjoying this diet.

Chapter 2: Heart-Healthy Savory Meals

Shrimp Scampi and Zoodles

Ingredients

- Butter (1 Tbsp., unsalted)
- Dry white wine (0.5 c.)
- Garlic (4 cloves, grated)
- Lemon juice (2 Tbsp.)
- Lemon zest (1 Tbsp.)
- Linguini (6 oz.)
- Olive oil (2 Tbsp.)
- Parsley (0.25 c., chopped)
- Red pepper flakes (0.25 tsp.)
- Shrimp (1.5 lbs., peeled and deveined—preferably large)
- Zucchini (3, spiralized)

Instructions

1. Start by preparing the pasta based on the instructions on the package. Keep 0.25 c. of the water to the side and drain the rest. Put pasta back in the pot.
2. Combine the shrimp, garlic, oil, salt, and pepper to taste and allow it to sit for five minutes.
3. Prepare a skillet and cook your shrimp in the garlicky oil over medium and garlic until done, roughly 3-4 minutes per side with a large count. Move shrimp to plate without the oil.
4. Add zest and pepper to the oil, along with the wine. Scrape the brown bits and reduce to 50%. Mix in lemon juice and butter, then toss the zoodles in.
5. After 2 minutes, add in shrimp, pasta, and combine well. Mix in water if necessary and toss with parsley.

Citrus Chicken Salad

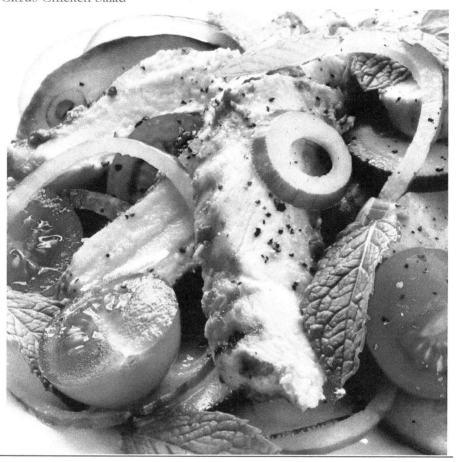

Ingredients

- Baby kale (5 oz.)
- Chicken thighs (2 lbs.)
- Dijon mustard (1 tsp)
- Lemon juice (2 Tbsp.)
- Olive oil (2 Tbsp.)
- Orange (1, cut into 6 pieces)
- Salt and pepper
- Stale bread (8 oz., torn up into bite-sized bits)

Instructions

1. Warm oven to 425F. As it preheats, warm up half of your oil into a skillet. Then, salt and pepper the chicken, cooking it skin-side down in the oil. After 6 or 7 minutes, when the skin is golden, remove it to a baking sheet. Then, toss in the orange wedges and roast another 10 minutes until the chicken is completely cooked.
2. Reserve 2 Tbsp. of the chicken fat in the pot and then return it to low heat. Toss in the bread chunks, coating them in the fat. Add a quick sprinkle of salt and pepper, then cook until toasted, usually about 8 minutes or so. Set aside.
3. Warm pan on medium-low, then toss in lemon juice. Deglaze the pan for a minute, then remove from heat. Combine with Dijon mustard and juice from roasted oranges. Mix in remaining oil.
4. Add kale and croutons to skillet to mix well, coating it in the mixture. Serve immediately with chicken.

Shrimp Taco Salad

Ingredients

- 3 Fresh lime juice (3 tbsp.)
- Avocado (1)
- Cayenne pepper sauce (1 tsp.)
- Cilantro leaves (1 c.)
- Corn chips (such as Fritos-- 2 c.)
- Extra-virgin olive oil (0.25 c.)
- Fresh corn (3 pieces)
- Ground coriander (0.25 tsp.)
- Ground cumin (0.25 tsp.)
- Salt
- Shrimp (1 lb.)
- Watermelon (2 c.)
- Zucchini (2 medium)

Instructions

1. Set up your grill to medium heat.
2. First grill the corn until it begins to char, usually about 10 minutes, with the occasional turn. At the same time, allow zucchini to grill for around 6 minutes until beginning to soften. Shrimp requires 2-4 minutes until cooked through, flipping once.
3. Combine your oil, juice, and seasonings, with just a pinch of salt.
4. Remove the kernels off of your corn and slice up your zucchini. Place zucchini and avocado onto a plate, topping it with the corn, then the watermelon, and finally the shrimp. You can leave it as is until you're ready to eat—it keeps for about a day in the fridge.
5. To serve, top with the chips (crumbled) and the dressing mix.

Chicken, Green Bean, Bacon Pasta

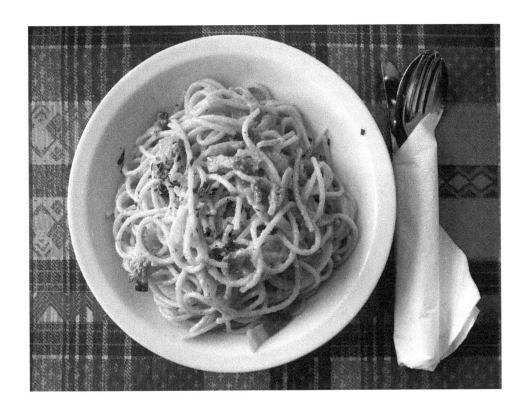

Ingredients

- Bacon (4 slices)
- Chicken breast (1 lb., cut into bite-sized bits)
- Egg yolk (1 large)
- Green beans (fresh—8 oz., trimmed and cut in half)
- Half-and-half (2 Tbsp.)
- Lemon juice (2 Tbsp.)
- Parmesan cheese (1 oz., grated—about 0.5 c.)
- Penne pasta (12 oz.)
- Scallions (2, sliced thinly)
- Spinach (5 oz.)

Instructions

1. Prepare pasta according to the package. Then, at the last minute of cooking, toss in the beans. Drain, reserving 0.5 c. of the cooking water. Leave pasta mix in the pot.
2. In a skillet, start preparing the bacon until crisp. Dry on a paper towel and then break into bits when cooled. Clean pan, reserving 1 Tbsp. of bacon fat.
3. On medium heat, cook the chicken until browning and cooked all the way. Then, off of the burner, toss in the lemon juice.
4. Mix together your egg and half-and-half in a separate container. Then, dump it to coat in the pasta and green beans, then toss in the chicken, spinach, and cheese. Mix well to coat. Add pasta water if needed, 0.25 c. at a time. Mix in the scallions, then top with bacon. Serve.

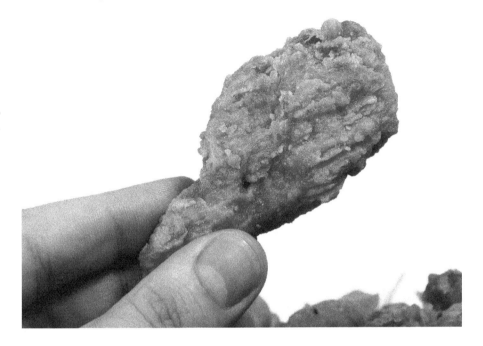

Ingredients

- Blackening seasoning (2 tsp.)
- Buttermilk (0.5 c.)
- Chicken drumsticks (2 lb., skinless)
- Cornflakes (4 c.)
- Olive oil (1 Tbsp.)
- Parsley (0.5 c., chopped)
- Salt (a pinch to taste)

Instructions

1. Get ready to bake the chicken at a temperature of 375F and make sure that you've got something to bake on that is currently protected.
2. Mix buttermilk, seasoning, and a touch of salt.
3. Crush cornflakes and put them in a second bowl. Combine with the oil and parsley.
4. Prep chicken by dipping first in buttermilk, letting it drip, then coating in cornflakes. Bake for 30-35 minutes.

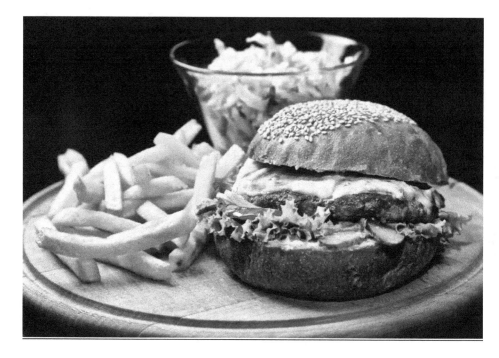

Ingredients

Slaw

- Apple (1, matchstick-cut)
- Cabbage (8 oz., thinly sliced)
- Honey (1 Tbsp.)
- Jalapeno (1, thinly sliced and seeded)
- Lime juice (3 Tbsp.)
- Red wine vinegar (1 Tbsp.)
- Salt and pepper, to your preference

Burgers

- Buns (4, toasted lightly)
- Chili paste (1.5 Tbsp.)
- Ginger (1 Tbsp., grated)
- Olive oil (2 Tbsp.)

- Onion (0.5 chopped)
- Soy sauce (1 Tbsp.)
- Turkey (1 lb., ground up)

Instructions

1. Mix together the liquids for the slaw and the seasoning. Mix well, then toss in the slaw ingredients. Set aside.
2. Prepare your burger mixture, adding everything together, but the oil and the buns somewhere that you can mix them up. Combine well, then form four patties.
3. Prepare to your preference. Grills work well, or you choose to, you could use a cast iron pan with the oil. Cook until done.
4. Serve on buns with slaw and any other condiments you may want.

Slow Cooked Shrimp and Pasta

Ingredients

- Acini di pepe (4 oz., cooked to package specifications)
- Basil (0.25 c., chopped fresh)
- Diced tomatoes (14.5 oz. can)
- Feta (2 oz., crumbled)
- Garlic (2 cloves, minced)
- Kalamata olives (8, chopped)
- Olive oil (1 Tbsp.)
- Pinch of salt
- Rosemary (1.5 tsp fresh, chopped)
- Shrimp (8 oz., fresh or frozen)
- Sweet red bell pepper (1, chopped)
- White wine (0.5 c.) or chicken broth (o.5 c.)
- Zucchini (1 c., sliced)

Instructions

1. Thaw, peel, and devein shrimp. Set aside in fridge until ready to use them.
2. Coat your slow cooker insert with cooking spray, then add in tomato, zucchini tomatoes, bell pepper, and garlic.
3. Cook on low for 4 hours, or high for 2 hours. Mix in shrimp. Then, keep heat on high. Cook covered for 30 minutes.
4. Prepare pasta according to the instructions on the packaging.
5. Mix in the olives, rosemary, basil, oil, and salt.
6. Serve with pasta topped with shrimp, then topped with feta.

Chapter 3: Heart-Healthy Sweet Treats

Chocolate Mousse

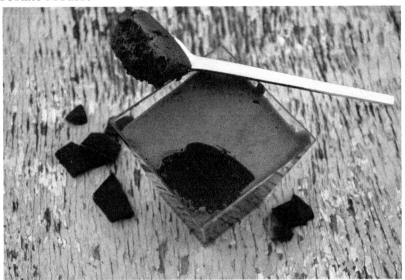

Ingredients

- Avocado (1 large, pitted and skinned)
- Cocoa powder (2 Tbsp., unsweetened)
- Nondairy milk of choice (3 Tbsp., unsweetened)
- Nonfat vanilla Greek yogurt (0.25 c.)
- Semi-sweet baking chocolate (2 oz., melted and cooling)
- Sweetener packet if desired.
- Vanilla extract (1 tsp.)

Instructions

1. Prepare by putting all ingredients but sugar into a food processor. Combine well. Taste. If you want it sweeter, add in some sweetener as well.
2. Chill in your fridge until you are ready to serve.

Baked Pears

Ingredients

- Almonds (0.25 c., chopped)
- Brown sugar (0.33 c., can sub with honey)
- Butter (2 oz., melted, or coconut oil if you prefer vegan)
- Ground cinnamon (1 tsp)
- Ripe pears (3)
- Rolled oats (0.5 c.)
- Salt (a pinch)
- Sugar (pinch)

Instructions

1. Set oven to 400 F.
2. Incorporate all dry ingredients. Then, mix half of your melted butter.
3. Cut your pears in half and carve out the cores, making a nice scoop in the center. Brush with butter, then top with a sprinkle of sugar.
4. Put your cinnamon oat mixture into the centers of the pears.
5. Bake for 30-40 minutes, until soft.

Chocolate Peanut Butter Bites

Ingredients

- Chocolate chips of choice (2 c.)
- Coconut flour (1 c.)
- Honey (0.75 c.)
- Smooth peanut butter (2 c.)

Instructions

1. Prepare a tray with parchment paper to avoid sticking or messes
2. Melt together your peanut butter and honey, mixing well
3. Add coconut flour to peanut butter mixture and combine to incorporate. If it's still thin, add small amounts of flour. Let it thicken for 10 minutes.
4. Create 20 balls out of the dough.
5. Melt chocolate, then dip the dough balls into the chocolate and place them on the parchment. Refrigerate until firm

Oatmeal Cookies

Ingredients

- Applesauce (2.5 Tbsp.)
- Baking soda (0.25 tsp)
- Coconut oil (2 Tbsp., melted)
- Dark chocolate chips (0.25 c.)
- Honey (0.25 c.)
- Salt (0.5 tsp)
- Vanilla extract (2 tsp.)
- Whole grain oats (0.5 c.)
- Whole wheat flour (0.5 c.)

Instructions

1. Set your oven to 350 F.
2. Mix syrup, oil (melted), applesauce, and vanilla.
3. Toss in salt, baking soda, oats, and flour. Combine well until it becomes a dough.
4. Mix the chocolate chips in.
5. Put in tablespoons onto cookie sheet.
6. Bake for 10 minutes. Let cool before transferring to a cooling rack.

Kiwi Sorbet

Ingredients

- Kiwi (1 lb., peeled and frozen)
- Honey (0.25 c.)

Instructions

1. Combine everything well in a food processor until mixed.
2. Pour it into a loaf pan and smooth it out.
3. Allow it to freeze for 2 hours. Keep it covered if leaving it overnight in the freezer.

Pina Colada Frozen Dessert

Ingredients

- Butter (0.25 c.)
- Crushed pineapple in juice (undrained—1 8 oz. can)
- Graham cracker crumbs (1.25 c.)
- Rum extract or rum (0.25 c.)
- Sugar (1 Tbsp.)
- Toasted flaked coconut (0.25 c.)
- Vanilla low-fat, no-sugar ice cream (4 c.)

Instructions

1. Prepare oven to 350 F.
2. Combine butter, cracker crumbs, and sugar. Press into a 2-quart baking dish. Bake 10 minutes and allow to cool completely
3. Combine ice cream, pineapple and juice, and extracts into a bowl with a mixer until well combined. Spread it out into the crust.
4. Freeze for 6 hours.
5. Serve after letting thaw for 5 minutes and topping with coconut shreds.

Ricotta Brûlée

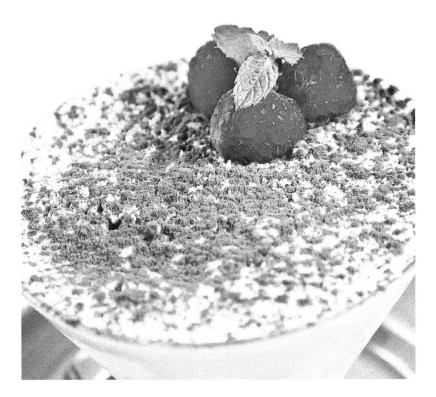

Ingredients

- Ricotta cheese (2 c.)
- Lemon zest (1 tsp)
- Honey (2 Tbsp.)
- Sugar (2 Tbsp.)

Instructions

1. Mix together your ricotta, lemon zest, and honey. Then, split into ramekins. Top with sugar and place onto baking sheet.
2. Place oven rack at the topmost position then set the baking sheet in with the broiler on its highest setting. Watch closely and broil until it bubbles and turns golden brown—between 5 and 10 minutes.
3. Cool for 10 minutes and top with any fruits or toppings you prefer.

Chapter 4: Heart-Healthy Gourmet Meals

Grilled Halibut With Pine Nut Relish

Ingredients

- Diced red tomato (0.5 c.)
- Diced yellow tomato (o.5 c)
- EVOO (3 Tbsp.)
- Flour to coat fish
- Green olives (0.5 c.)
- Halibut fillet (4, 1 inch thick)
- Kalamata olives (0.5 c.)
- Lemon juice (1 Tbsp.)
- Zest from a lemon (0.5 tsp.)
- Parsley (2 Tbsp.)
- Pepper to taste
- Pine nuts (3 Tbsp.)
- Salt (pinch to taste)
- Shallot (1)

Instructions

1. Start with toasting the pine nuts in a dry skillet for a few minutes until toasted. Set aside.
2. Combine your tomatoes, the sliced olives, shallot, the lemon juice and zest, and 1 Tbsp. of oil. Mix well and add in parsley and a sprinkle of pepper.
3. Flour fillets, shaking off excess. Season lightly with salt and pepper. Toss the rest of your oil into your skillet and use that to cook the fish until done, flipping halfway over.
4. Serve with relish on top and garnish with pine nuts.

Shrimp Bowls

Ingredients

- Avocado (1, cut small)
- Broccoli (1 lb., florets)
- Ginger (1 Tbsp.)
- Olive oil (2 Tbsp.)
- Plum tomatoes (8 oz., seeds removed and cut)
- Quinoa (1.5 c.)
- Rice vinegar (1 Tbsp.)
- Salt and pepper to taste
- Scallions (2, thinly sliced)
- Shrimp (20 large, peeled and deveined)

Instructions

1. Warm oven to 425 F. Prepare medium saucepan at medium heat and cook the quinoa until toasted, roughly 5 minutes. Add in water (3 c.), then cover immediately. Allow it to cook just below a boil for 10 minutes, then take it off the burner and let it sit for another ten minutes.
2. On a baking sheet, add broccoli, 1 Tbsp. oil, salt, and pepper. Prepare in a single layer. Roast for 15 minutes. Season shrimp, then cook for 6-8 minutes, tossed with broccoli.
3. Mix vinegar, ginger, and remaining oil into a small bowl. Toss with tomatoes and scallions.
4. Serve with quinoa in bowls, topped with broccoli shrimp, then avocado. Finally, add the vinaigrette to the top.

Grilled Watermelon Steak Salad

Ingredients

- Cherry tomatoes (1 lb., halved)
- Honey (1 tsp)
- Lemon juice (3 Tbsp.)
- Mint leaves (1 c., torn up)
- Olive oil (2 Tbsp.)
- Onion (0.5 tsp., small red)
- Parsley (1 c., chopped)
- Salt and pepper
- Sirloin steak (1 lb.)
- Unsalted peanuts to garnish
- Watermelon (3 lbs., seedless)

Instructions

1. Prepare grill to medium-high. Season steak, then grill until done to preference. Allow it to rest on a cutting board.
2. Mix oil, lemon juice, honey, and seasonings. Incorporate the onions and tomatoes as well, folding in nicely.
3. Cut watermelon into 0.5-inch thick triangles and remove rinds. Oil and grill until starting to char—a minute per side, then set aside.
4. Mix the herbs into the tomato mixture. Serve with watermelon topped with stead.

Crispy Cod and Green Beans

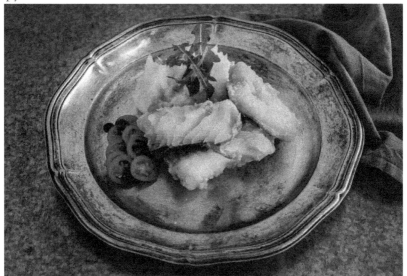

Ingredients

- Green Beans (1 lb.)
- Olive oil (2 Tbsp.)
- Parmesan cheese (0.25 c., grated)
- Pepper to taste
- Pesto (2 Tbsp.)
- Salt to taste
- Skinless cod (1.25 lb., four pieces)

Instructions

1. Set oven to 425 F. Put beans onto rimmed baking sheet and combine with 1 Tbsp. oil, then top with cheese and a sprinkling of seasonings. Roast for 10-12 minutes, waiting for it to finally start to brown.
2. Heat remaining oil in a skillet. Season cod and cook until golden brown. You want to use a medium-high heat to do this.
3. Serve with pesto over cod, next to a bed of green beans.

Pistachio-Crusted Fish

Ingredients

- Baby spinach (4 c.)
- Greek yogurt (4 Tbsp.)
- Lemon juice (2 Tbsp.)
- Olive oil (2 Tbsp.)
- Panko (whole-wheat, 0.25 c.)
- Pepper (0.5 tsp)
- Quinoa (0.75 c.)
- Salt (0.75 tsp)
- Shelled pistachios, chopped (0.25 c.)
- Tilapia (4 6-oz. pieces)

Instructions

1. Prepare quinoa based on instructions on packaging.
2. Season fish with salt, pepper, and coat with 1 Tbsp. each of Greek yogurt.
3. Combine panko and pistachios, tossing with 1 Tbsp. olive oil. Gently sprinkle over the top of the fish, pressing it to stick. Bake for 12 minutes at 375 F., or until done.
4. Combine cooked quinoa with spinach, lemon juice, remaining oil, and a pinch of salt and pepper. Serve with fish.

Cumin-Spiced Lamb and Salad

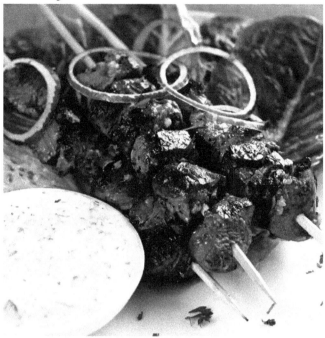

Ingredients

- Carrots (1 lb.)
- Cumin (1.25 tsp.)
- Honey (0.5 tsp.)
- Lamb loin chops (8—about 2 lbs.)
- Mint leaves (0.25 c., fresh)
- Olive oil (3 Tbsp.)
- Radishes (6)
- Red wine vinegar (2 Tbsp.)
- Salt and pepper to taste

Instructions

1. Combine 2 Tbsp. oil, vinegar, a pinch of cumin, honey, and salt and pepper.
2. Warm remaining oil in a skillet at medium. Season lamb with cumin and a pinch of salt and pepper. Cook until preferred doneness.
3. Shave carrots into pieces and create thinly sliced radishes. Coat with dressing and mix with mint. Serve with lamb.

Chapter 5: Heart-Healthy Quick 'n Easy Meals

Sugar Snap Pea and Radish Salad

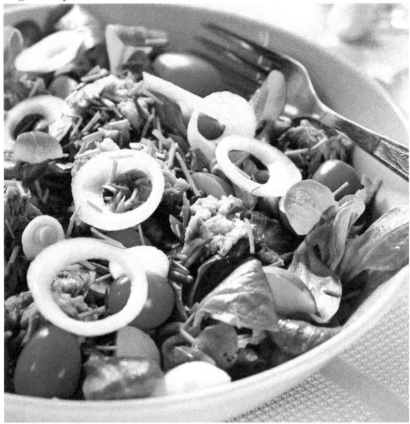

Ingredients

- Apple-cider vinegar (2 Tbsp.)
- Avocado (0.5, medium ripe)
- Dijon mustard (0.5 tsp)
- Fresh lemon juice (1 Tbsp.)
- Freshly ground pepper (0.5 tsp)
- Ground coriander (0.25 tsp)

- Olive oil (0.25 c.)
- Radishes (12, small)
- Salt (o.5 tsp)
- Sugar snap peas (1 lb.)
- Watermelon radish (1, small)

Instructions

1. Combine peas and radishes in a bowl together.
2. In a blender, combine everything else and puree until well combined and smooth. Add water if necessary to thin it out.
3. Coat radish and peas with dressing and serve.

Horseradish Salmon Cakes

Ingredients

- Dijon mustard (1 Tbsp.)
- English cucumber (1, small)
- Greek Yogurt (2 Tbsp.)
- Horseradish (2 Tbsp.)
- Lemon juice (1 Tbsp.)
- Olive oil (2 Tbsp.)
- Panko (0.25 c.)
- Salt and pepper to taste
- Skinless salmon filet (1.25 lb.)
- Watercress (1 bunch)

Instructions

1. Combine salmon, horseradish, salt and pepper, and mustard into a food processor until well chopped. Then, toss in the bread crumbs and combine well.
2. Form 8 patties.
3. Warm 1 Tbsp. oil in a skillet. Cook until opaque throughout, typically 2 minutes before flipping.
4. Combine yogurt, lemon juice, oil, and a sprinkle of salt and pepper. Combine in cucumber slices, then watercress.
5. Serve salmon with salad.

Salmon, Green Beans, and Tomatoes

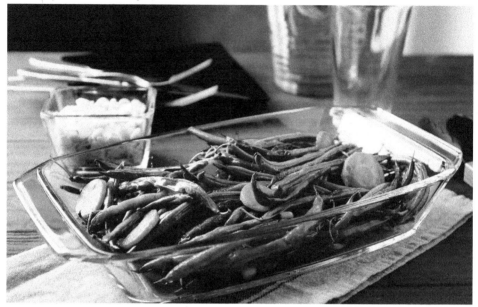

Ingredients

- Garlic (6 cloves)
- Green beans (1 lb.)
- Grape tomatoes (1 pint)
- Kalamata olives (0.5 c.)
- Anchovy fillets (3)
- Olive oil (2 Tbsp.)
- Kosher salt and pepper to personal preference
- Salmon fillet, skinless

Instructions

1. Prepare oven to 425 F. Put beans, garlic, olive, anchovy, and tomatoes together along with half of the oil and a pinch of pepper. Roast until veggies are tender.
2. Warm the remainder of the oil over a skillet at medium heat. Season salmon, then cook until done. Serve salmon and veggies together.

Broccoli Pesto Fusilli
Ingredients

- Basil leaves (0.5 c.)
- Broccoli florets (12 oz.)
- Fusilli (12 oz.)
- Garlic (2 cloves)
- Lemon zest (1 Tbsp.)
- Olive oil (3 Tbsp.)
- Parmesan cheese to garnish
- Salt to taste
- Sliced almonds to garnish

Instructions

1. Prepare pasta to directions and reserve 0.5 c. of the liquid.
2. Combine broccoli, garlic, and the reserved water in a bowl and cook for five or six minutes, stirring halfway through. Put everything right into a food processor with the liquid. Combine in basil, oil, zest, a pinch of salt, and puree.
3. Put pasta in with pesto. Drizzle in water if necessary. Sprinkle with cheese and nuts if desired. Serve immediately.

Strawberry Spinach Salad

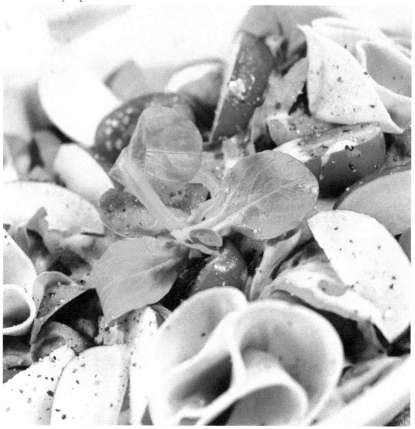

Ingredients

- Baby spinach (3 c.)
- Medium avocado (0.25, diced)
- Red onion (1 Tbsp.)
- Sliced strawberries (0.5 c.)
- Vinaigrette of choice (2 Tbsp.)
- Walnut pieces (roasted)

Instructions

1. Combine spinach with the berries and onion. Mix well. Coat with vinaigrette and toss. Then, top with walnuts and avocado. Serve.

Ingredients

- Crushed red pepper (0.25 tsp)
- Garlic (6 cloves, sliced)
- Lemon juice (1 Tbsp.)
- Lemon zest (1.5 tsp.)
- Olive oil (3 Tbsp.)
- Parsley (1 Tbsp.)
- Salt to personal preference
- Shrimp (1 lb.)
- Spinach (1 lb.)

Instructions

1. Warm skillet with 1 Tbsp. oil. Cook half of the garlic until browning, about a single minute. Then, toss in spinach and salt. Wait for it to wilt over the heat, about 5 minutes. Remove and mix in lemon juice, storing it in a separate bowl.
2. Warm heat to medium-high and toss with remainder of oil. Toss in the rest of your garlic and cook until browning. Then, mix in shrimp, pepper, and salt. Cook until shrimp is done, then serve atop spinach with lemon zest and parsley garnish.

Chapter 6: Heart-Healthy Vegetarian and Vegan Meals

Vegetarian Butternut Squash Torte
Ingredients

- Butternut squash (1 lb.)
- Crusty bread of choice
- Kale (1, small)
- Olive oil (1 Tbsp.)
- Parmesan cheese (4 Tbsp., grated)
- Plum tomato (1)
- Provolone cheese (6 oz., thinly sliced)
- Red onion (1, medium)
- Salt and pepper to taste
- Yukon Gold potato (1, medium)

Instructions

1. Take a spring form 9-inch pan and prepare it so that nothing will stick. Then, take your squash and put it around the bottom in circles to sort of mimic a crust.
2. Then, layer it with the onion, with the rings separated out.
3. Add half of your kale, then sprinkle half of your oil, and season to taste.
4. Then, layer with potatoes, half of your cheese, and top with the last of your kale.
5. Add the oil, onion, tomato slices, and the last of your cheese.
6. Top it with the remainder of your squash, then coat with parmesan.
7. Bake, covering the top with foil, for 20 minutes. Then, discard the foil and let it bake until it is tender and browning, typically another ten minutes or so.

Vegetarian Fried Rice
Ingredients

- 2 eggs (leave out if vegan)
- Garlic (2 cloves, pressed)
- Kale (6 oz., thinly sliced leaves)
- Olive oil (1 Tbsp.)
- Rice (4 c., cooked and chilled, preferably the day before)
- Sesame oil (1 Tbsp.)
- Shiitake mushroom caps (4 oz., sliced)
- Soy sauce (2 Tbsp., low sodium)
- Sriracha (1 tsp.)

Instructions

1. Start by warming your oil up in your pan of choice or wok. Your oil should be just before the smoking point.
2. Cook the mushrooms and toss until they start to turn golden brown, usually just a few minutes, then set them off for later.
3. Toss in some sesame oil and kale, cooking until wilted, then add in your garlic as well for another minute.
4. Take your rice and mix it in as well, tossing it together until heated.
5. Move all rice to the side, then pour beaten eggs in the center of your pan. Stir often until the eggs are just about finished, and then mix into the rice.
6. Mix in the soy sauce and sriracha, then top with mushrooms.

Vegan Butternut Squash Soup

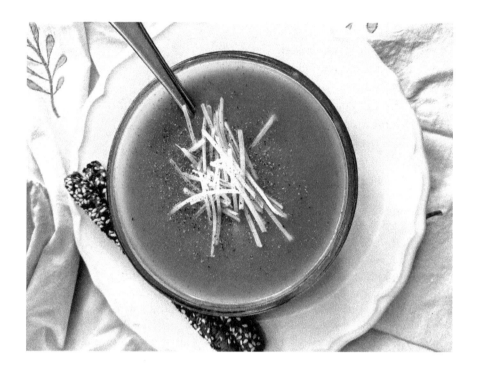

Ingredients

- Butternut squash (1, 2.5 lbs. with skin and seeds removed—keep seeds)
- Carrots (2 medium, cut into 1-inch pieces)
- Coconut milk (2 Tbsp.)
- Olive oil (2 Tbsp., and one tsp)
- Onion (1, large, chopped)
- Pepper (2.25 tsp)
- Turmeric (2.25 tsp)
- Veggie bouillon base (1 Tbsp.)

Instructions

1. Take a Dutch oven and add 2 Tbsp. oil. Warm, then cook your onions until soft and translucent, roughly 6 minutes or so.

2. Integrate your bouillon base with 6 c., boiling water until completely dissolved.
3. Toss together your veggies, turmeric, and pepper into your onions in the Dutch oven. Allow it to cook for a minute before mixing in your veggie broth. Simmer for 20 minutes until veggies are soft.
4. Turn your oven to 375F. Take your seeds and your oil that is remaining and combine them together. Then, coat it up with the turmeric and pepper before toasting in your oven for about 1o minutes.
5. With a blender or immersion blender, combine your soup until smooth.
6. Serve topped with seeds and a swirl of coconut milk.

Vegetarian Kale and Sweet Potato Frittata

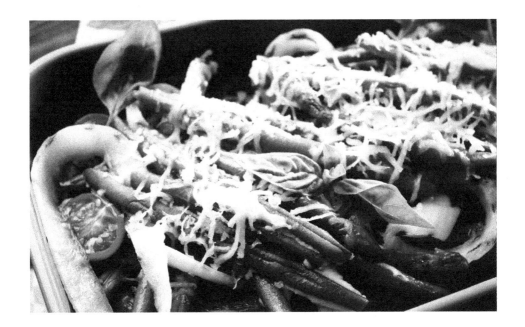

Ingredients

- Eggs (6)
- Garlic (2 cloves)
- Goat cheese (3 oz.)
- Half-and-half (1 c.)

- Kale (2 c., packed tightly)
- Olive oil (2 Tbsp.)
- Pepper (0.5 tsp.)
- Red onion (0.5, small)
- Salt (1 tsp.)
- Sweet potatoes (2 c.)

Instructions

1. With your oven warming, combine your eggs in a bowl. Then, add in the salt and half-and-half as well. Make sure your oven is at 350F.
2. In a nonstick skillet that you can put into your oven, cook your potatoes over 1 Tbsp. of oil. Wait for them to soften and start to turn golden. Then, remove from the pan.
3. Next, cook your kale, onion, and garlic together in the remainder of your oil until it is wilted and aromatic.
4. Put your potato back in with the kale, then pour your egg mix atop it all. Incorporate well and then allow it to cook on the stove for another 3 minutes.
5. Top it all with the goat cheese, then bake for 10 minutes until completely done.

Vegan Ginger Ramen
Ingredients

- Garlic (4 cloves, minced)
- Ginger (0.33 c., chopped coarsely)
- Grapeseed oil (0.5 c.)
- Low-sodium soy sauce (2 Tbsp.)
- Pepper (1 tsp., freshly ground)
- Ramen noodles (*real,* fresh noodles—not the $0.10 packaged stuff)
- Rice vinegar (1 Tbsp.)
- Salt to personal preference
- Scallions (1 bunch—about 2 c. sliced)
- Sesame oil (1 tsp)
- Sugar (0.5 tsp)

Instructions

1. Combine your ginger with the minced garlic and roughly 60% of your scallions.
2. Warm up the grapeseed oil until just before the smoking point. Then, take the oil and dump it over your scallion mix. It will sizzle and wilt, turning green. Leave it for 5 minutes, then add in the rest of the scallions.
3. Carefully combine in soy sauce, sesame oil, vinegar, sugar, and pepper, and leave it to incorporate for the next 15 minutes or so. Adjust flavor accordingly.
4. Prepare your noodles to the package instructions. Drain.
5. Introduce your noodles to your scallion sauce and coat well.
6. Serve topped with sesame seeds or any other toppings you may want.

Vegan Glazed Tofu

Ingredients

- Canola oil (0.5 c.)
- Firm tofu (12 oz.)
- Ginger (0.5" sliced thinly)
- Maple syrup (3 Tbsp.—you can use honey if you're not vegan.)
- Pepper flakes (0.5 tsp.)
- Rice vinegar (3 Tbsp.)
- Soy sauce (4 Tbsp.)
- Toppings of choice—recommended ones include rice, scallions, or sesame seeds

Instructions

1. Dry and drain your tofu out, squeezing it between paper towels so that you can remove as much of the liquid as you possibly can, then slice it into cubes.
2. Combine the wet ingredients together, and add in your pepper and ginger.
3. Warm your wok or skillet. When the oil is shimmery, gingerly place your tofu into it carefully and leave it for around 4 minutes so that it can brown. It should be dark brown when you flip. Repeat on both sides. Then, drop the heat down and toss in your sauce mix. Allow it to reduce until it is thick, roughly 4 minutes.
4. Put tofu on plates and top with anything you desire.

Vegan Greek Tofu Breakfast Scramble

Ingredients

- Basil (0.25 c., chopped)
- Firm tofu block (8 oz.)
- Garlic (2 cloves, diced)
- Grape tomatoes (0.5 c., halved)
- Kalamata olives (0.25 c., halved)
- Lemon juice (from ½ lemon)
- Nutritional yeast (2 Tbsp.)
- Olive oil (1 Tbsp.)
- Red bell pepper (0.5 c., chopped)
- Red onion (0.25, diced)
- Salt (pinch)
- Spinach (1 handful)
- Tahini paste (1 tsp)
- Salt and pepper to personal preference

Instructions

1. Break down tofu until the shape/texture of scrambled eggs. Then, combine in yeast, lemon juice, and tahini. Sprinkle with a pinch of salt.
2. Prepare skillet at a moderate heat. Sauté onions for 5 minutes before tossing in the pepper and garlic for an additional 5 minutes.
3. Mix in tofu and Kalamata olives. Warm through.
4. Toss in greens until wilted and reduced. Take off from heat and toss in tomatoes and season with salt and pepper to taste.

PART II

Smoothie Diet Recipes

The smoothie diet is all about replacing some of your meals with smoothies that are loaded with veggies and fruits. It has been found that the smoothie diet is very helpful in losing weight along with excess fat. The ingredients of the smoothies will vary, but they will focus mainly on vegetables and fruits. The best part about the smoothie diet is that there is no need to count your calorie intake and less food tracking. The diet is very low in calories and is also loaded with phytonutrients.

Apart from weight loss, there are various other benefits of the smoothie diet. It can help you to stay full for a longer time as most smoothies are rich in fiber. It can also help you to control your cravings as smoothies are full of flavor and nutrients. Whenever you feel like snacking, just prepare a smoothie, and you are good to go. Also, smoothies can aid in digestion as they are rich in important minerals and vitamins. Fruits such as mango are rich in carotenoids that can help in improving your skin quality. As the smoothie diet is mainly based on veggies and fruits, it can detoxify your body.

In this section, you will find various recipes of smoothies that you can include in your smoothie diet.

Chapter 1: Fruit Smoothies

The best way of having fruits is by making smoothies. Fruit smoothies can help you start your day with loads of nutrients so that you can remain energetic throughout the day. Here are some easy-to-make fruit smoothie recipes that you can enjoy during any time of the day.

Quick Fruit Smoothie

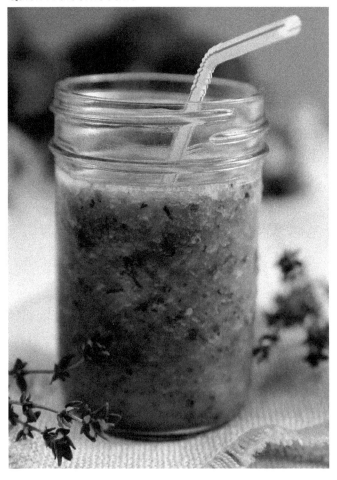

Total Prep & Cooking Time: Fifteen minutes

Yields: Four servings

Nutrition Facts: Calories: 115.2 | Protein: 1.2g | Carbs: 27.2g | Fat: 0.5g | Fiber: 3.6g

Ingredients

- One cup of strawberries
- One banana (cut in chunks)
- Two peaches
- Two cups of ice
- One cup of orange and mango juice

Method:

1. Add banana, strawberries, and peaches in a blender.

2. Blend until frothy and smooth.

3. Add the orange and mango juice and blend again. Add ice for adjusting the consistency and blend for two minutes.

4. Divide the smoothie in glasses and serve with mango chunks from the top.

Triple Threat Smoothie

Total Prep & Cooking Time: Ten minutes

Yields: Four servings

Nutrition Facts: Calories: 132.2 | Protein: 3.4g | Carbs: 27.6g | Fat: 1.3g | Fiber: 2.7g

Ingredients

- One kiwi (sliced)
- One banana (chopped)
- One cup of each
    - Ice cubes
    - Strawberries
- Half cup of blueberries
- One-third cup of orange juice
- Eight ounces of peach yogurt

Method:

1. Add kiwi, strawberries, and bananas in a food processor.

2. Blend until smooth.

3. Add the blueberries along with orange juice. Blend again for two minutes.

4. Add peach yogurt and ice cubes. Give it a pulse.

5. Pour the prepared smoothie in smoothie glasses and serve with blueberry chunks from the top.

Tropical Smoothie

Total Prep & Cooking Time: Fifteen minutes

Yields: Two servings

Nutrition Facts: Calories: 127.3 | Protein: 1.6g | Carbs: 30.5g | Fat: 0.7g | Fiber: 4.2g

Ingredients

- One mango (seeded)
- One papaya (cubed)
- Half cup of strawberries
- One-third cup of orange juice
- Five ice cubes

Method:

1. Add mango, strawberries, and papaya in a blender. Blend the ingredients until smooth.

2. Add ice cubes and orange juice for adjusting the consistency.

3. Blend again.

4. Serve with strawberry chunks from the top.

Fruit and Mint Smoothie

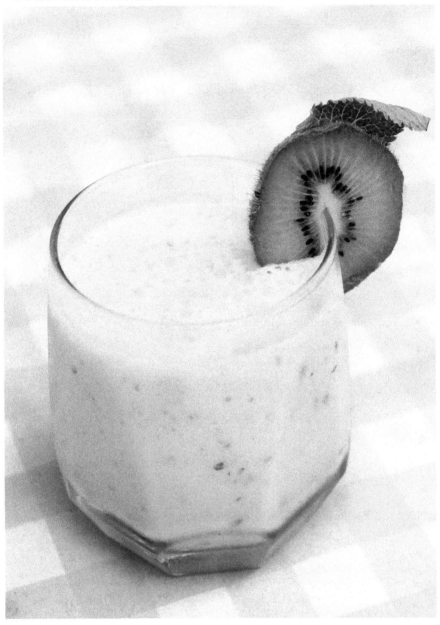

Total Prep & Cooking Time: Fifteen minutes

Yields: Two servings

Nutrition Facts: Calories: 90.3 | Protein: 0.7g | Carbs: 21.4g | Fat: 0.4g | Fiber: 2.5g

Ingredients

- One-fourth cup of each
    - Applesauce (unsweetened)
    - Red grapes (seedless, frozen)
- One tbsp. of lime juice
- Three strawberries (frozen)
- One cup of pineapple cubes
- Three mint leaves

Method:

1. Add grapes, lime juice, and applesauce in a blender. Blend the ingredients until frothy and smooth.

2. Add pineapple cubes, mint leaves, and frozen strawberries in the blender. Pulse the ingredients for a few times until the pineapple and strawberries are crushed.

3. Serve with mint leaves from the top.

Banana Smoothie

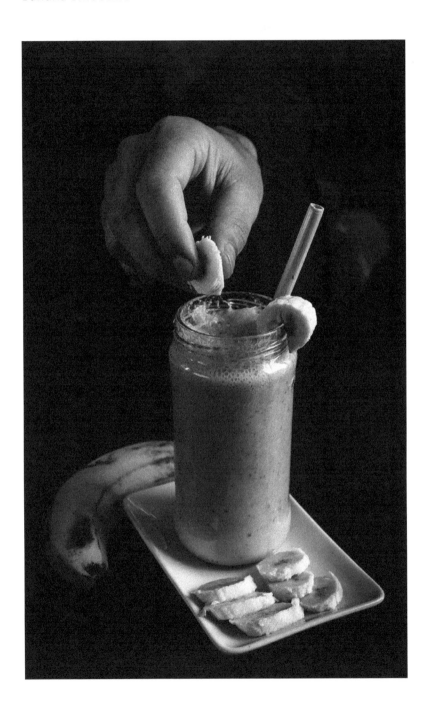

Total Prep & Cooking Time: Ten minutes

Yields: Four servings

Nutrition Facts: Calories: 122.6 | Protein: 1.3g | Carbs: 34.6g | Fat: 0.4g | Fiber: 2.2g

Ingredients

- Three bananas (sliced)
- One cup of fresh pineapple juice
- One tbsp. of honey
- Eight cubes of ice

Method:

1. Combine the bananas and pineapple juice in a blender.

2. Blend until smooth.

3. Add ice cubes along with honey.

4. Blend for two minutes.

5. Serve immediately.

Dragon Fruit Smoothie

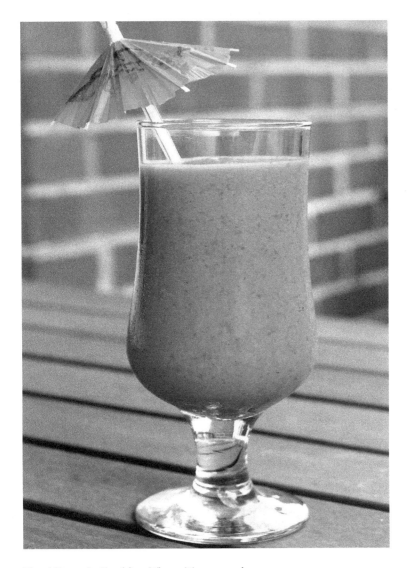

Total Prep & Cooking Time: Twenty minutes

Yields: Four servings

Nutrition Facts: Calories: 147.6 | Protein: 5.2g | Carbs: 21.4g | Fat: 6.4g | Fiber: 2.9g

Ingredients

- One-fourth cup of almonds
- Two tbsps. of shredded coconut
- One tsp. of chocolate chips
- One cup of yogurt
- One dragon fruit (chopped)
- Half cup of pineapple cubes
- One tbsp. of honey

Method:

1. Add almonds, dragon fruit, coconut, and chocolate chips in a high power blender. Blend until smooth.

2. Add yogurt, pineapple, and honey. Blend well.

3. Serve with chunks of dragon fruit from the top.

Kefir Blueberry Smoothie

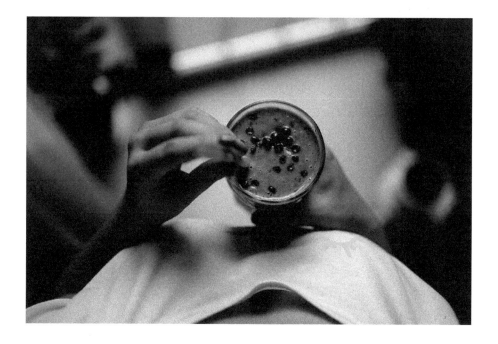

Total Prep & Cooking Time: Fifteen minutes

Yields: Two servings

Nutrition Facts: Calories: 304.2 | Protein: 7.3g | Carbs: 41.3g | Fat: 13.2g | Fiber: 4.6g

Ingredients

- Half cup of kefir
- One cup of blueberries (frozen)
- Half banana (cubed)

- One tbsp. of almond butter
- Two tsps. of honey

Method:

1. Add blueberries, banana cubes, and kefir in a blender.

2. Blend until smooth.

3. Add honey and almond butter.

4. Pulse the smoothie for a few times.

5. Serve immediately.

Ginger Fruit Smoothie

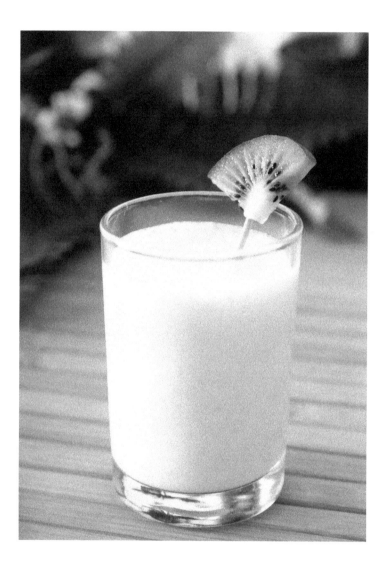

Total Prep & Cooking Time: Fifteen minutes

Yields: Two servings

Nutrition Facts: Calories: 160.2 | Protein: 1.9g | Carbs: 41.3g | Fat: 0.7g | Fiber: 5.6g

Ingredients

- One-fourth cup of each
    - Blueberries (frozen)
    - Green grapes (seedless)
- Half cup of green apple (chopped)
- One cup of water
- Three strawberries
- One piece of ginger
- One tbsp. of agave nectar

Method:

1. Add blueberries, grapes, and water in a blender. Blend the ingredients.

2. Add green apple, strawberries, agave nectar, and ginger. Blend for making thick slushy.

3. Serve immediately.

Fruit Batido

Total Prep & Cooking Time: Fifteen minutes

Yields: Six servings

Nutrition Facts: Calories: 129.3 | Protein: 4.2g | Carbs: 17.6g | Fat: 4.6g | Fiber: 0.6g

Ingredients

- One can of evaporated milk
- One cup of papaya (chopped)
- One-fourth cup of white sugar
- One tsp. of vanilla extract
- One tsp. of cinnamon (ground)
- One tray of ice cubes

Method:

1. Add papaya, white sugar, cinnamon, and vanilla extract in a food processor. Blend the ingredients until smooth.

2. Add milk and ice cubes. Blend for making slushy.

3. Serve immediately.

Banana Peanut Butter Smoothie

Total Prep & Cooking Time: Ten minutes

Yields: Four servings

Nutrition Facts: Calories: 332 | Protein: 13.2g | Carbs: 35.3g | Fat: 17.8g | Fiber: 3.9g

Ingredients

- Two bananas (cubed)
- Two cups of milk
- Half cup of peanut butter
- Two tbsps. of honey
- Two cups of ice cubes

Method:

1. Add banana cubes and peanut butter in a blender. Blend for making a smooth paste.

2. Add milk, ice cubes, and honey. Blend the ingredients until smooth.

3. Serve with banana chunks from the top.

Chapter 2: Breakfast Smoothies

Smoothie forms an essential part of breakfast in the smoothie diet plan. Here are some breakfast smoothie recipes for you that can be included in your daily breakfast plan.

Berry Banana Smoothie

Total Prep & Cooking Time: Twenty minutes

Yields: Two servings

Nutrition Facts: Calories: 330 | Protein: 6.7g | Carbs: 56.3g | Fat: 13.2g | Fiber: 5.5g

Ingredients

- One cup of each
  - Strawberries
  - Peaches (cubed)
  - Apples (cubed)
- One banana (cubed)
- Two cups of vanilla ice cream
- Half cup of ice cubes
- One-third cup of milk

Method:

1. Place strawberries, peaches, banana, and apples in a blender. Pulse the ingredients.

2. Add milk, ice cream, and ice cubes. Blend the smoothie until frothy and smooth.

3. Serve with a scoop of ice cream from the top.

Berry Surprise

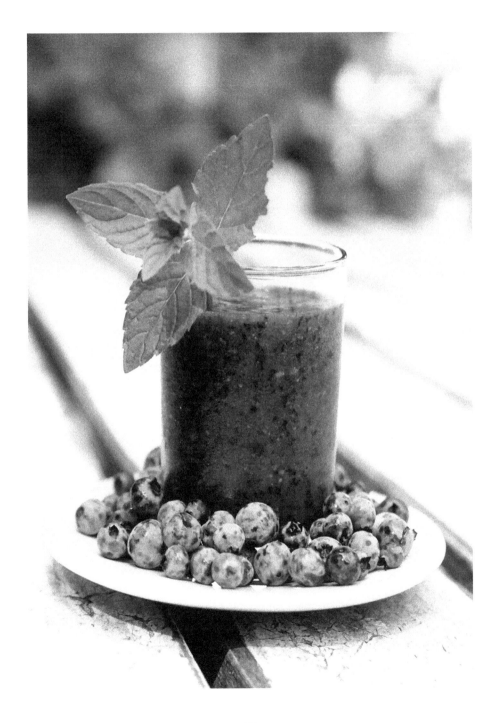

Total Prep & Cooking Time: Ten minutes

Yields: Two servings

Nutrition Facts: Calories: 164.2 | Protein: 1.2g | Carbs: 40.2g | Fat: 0.4g | Fiber: 4.8g

Ingredients

- One cup of strawberries
- Half cup of pineapple cubes
- One-third cup of raspberries
- Two tbsps. of limeade concentrate (frozen)

Method:

1. Combine pineapple cubes, strawberries, and raspberries in a food processor. Blend the ingredients until smooth.

2. Add the frozen limeade and blend again.

3. Divide the smoothie in glasses and serve immediately.

Coconut Matcha Smoothie

Total Prep & Cooking Time: Twenty minutes

Yields: Two servings

Nutrition Facts: Calories: 362 | Protein: 7.2g | Carbs: 70.1g | Fat: 8.7g | Fiber: 12.1g

Ingredients

- One large banana
- One cup of frozen mango cubes
- Two leaves of kale (torn)
- Three tbsps. of white beans (drained)
- Two tbsps. of shredded coconut (unsweetened)
- Half tsp. of matcha green tea (powder)
- Half cup of water

Method:

1. Add cubes of mango, banana, white beans, and kale in a blender. Blend all the ingredients until frothy and smooth.

2. Add shredded coconut, white beans, water, and green tea powder. Blend for thirty seconds.

3. Serve with shredded coconut from the top.

Cantaloupe Frenzy

Total Prep & Cooking Time: Ten minutes

Yields: Three servings

Nutrition Facts: Calories: 108.3 | Protein: 1.6g | Carbs: 26.2g | Fat: 0.2g | Fiber: 1.6g

Ingredients

- One cantaloupe (seeded, chopped)
- Three tbsps. of white sugar
- Two cups of ice cubes

Method:

1. Place the chopped cantaloupe along with white sugar in a blender. Puree the mixture.

2. Add cubes of ice and blend again.

3. Pour the smoothie in serving glasses. Serve immediately.

Berry Lemon Smoothie

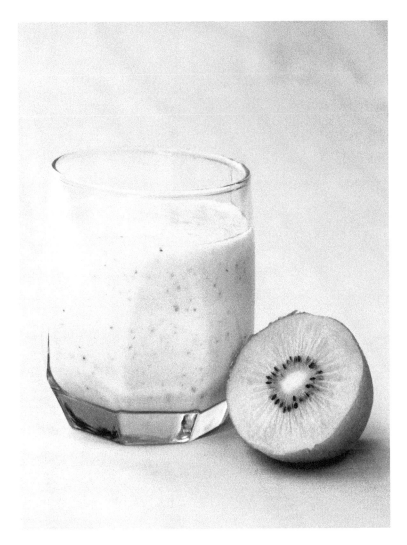

Total Prep & Cooking Time: Ten minutes

Yields: Four servings

Nutrition Facts: Calories: 97.2 | Protein: 5.4g | Carbs: 19.4g | Fat: 0.4g | Fiber: 1.8g

Ingredients

- Eight ounces of blueberry yogurt
- One and a half cup of milk (skim)
- One cup of ice cubes
- Half cup of blueberries
- One-third cup of strawberries
- One tsp. of lemonade mix

Method:

1. Add blueberry yogurt, skim milk, blueberries, and strawberries in a food processor. Blend the ingredients until smooth.

2. Add lemonade mix and ice cubes. Pulse the mixture for making a creamy and smooth smoothie.

3. Divide the smoothie in glasses and serve.

Orange Glorious

Total Prep & Cooking Time: Ten minutes

Yields: Four servings

Nutrition Facts: Calories: 212 | Protein: 3.4g | Carbs: 47.3g | Fat: 1.5g | Fiber: 0.5g

Ingredients

- Six ounces of orange juice concentrate (frozen)
- One cup of each
  - Water
  - Milk
- Half cup of white sugar
- Twelve ice cubes
- One tsp. of vanilla extract

Method:

1. Combine orange juice concentrate, white sugar, milk, and water in a blender.

2. Add vanilla extract and ice cubes. Blend the mixture until smooth.

3. Pour the smoothie in glasses and enjoy!

Grapefruit Smoothie

Total Prep & Cooking Time: Ten minutes

Yields: Two servings

Nutrition Facts: Calories: 200.3 | Protein: 4.7g | Carbs: 46.3g | Fat: 1.2g | Fiber: 7.6g

Ingredients

- Three grapefruits (peeled)
- One cup of water
- Three ounces of spinach
- Six ice cubes
- Half-inch piece of ginger
- One tsp. of flax seeds

Method:

1. Combine spinach, grapefruit, and ginger in a high power blender. Blend until smooth.

2. Add water, flax seeds, and ice cubes. Blend smooth.

3. Pour the smoothie in glasses and serve.

Sour Smoothie

Total Prep & Cooking Time: Ten minutes

Yields: Two servings

Nutrition Facts: Calories: 102.6 | Protein: 2.3g | Carbs: 30.2g | Fat: 0.7g | Fiber: 7.9g

Ingredients

- One cup of ice cubes
- Two fruit limes (peeled)
- One orange (peeled)
- One lemon (peeled)
- One kiwi (peeled)
- One tsp. of honey

Method:

1. Add fruit limes, lemon, orange, and kiwi in a food processor. Blend until frothy and smooth.

2. Add cubes of ice and honey. Pulse the ingredients.

3. Divide the smoothie in glasses and enjoy!

Ginger Orange Smoothie
Total Prep & Cooking Time: Ten minutes

Yields: One serving

Nutrition Facts: Calories: 115.6 | Protein: 2.2g | Carbs: 27.6g | Fat: 1.3g | Fiber: 5.7g

Ingredients

- One large orange
- Two carrots (peeled, cut in chunks)
- Half cup of each
    - Red grapes
    - Ice cubes
- One-fourth cup of water
- One-inch piece of ginger

Method:

1. Combine carrots, grapes, and orange in a high power blender. Blend until frothy and smooth.

2. Add ice cubes, ginger, and water. Blend the ingredients for thirty seconds.

3. Serve immediately.

Cranberry Smoothie

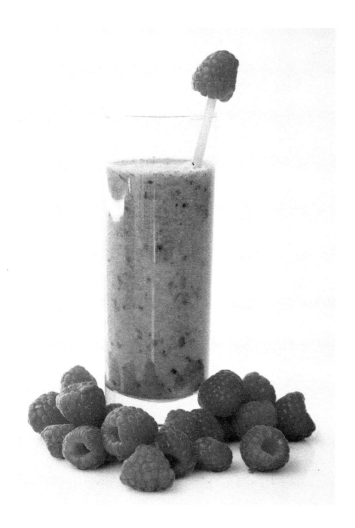

Total Prep & Cooking Time: One hour and ten minutes

Yields: Two servings

Nutrition Facts: Calories: 155.9 | Protein: 2.2g | Carbs: 33.8g | Fat: 1.6g | Fiber: 5.2g

Ingredients

- One cup of almond milk
- Half cup of mixed berries (frozen)
- One-third cup of cranberries
- One banana

Method:

1. Blend mixed berries, banana, and cranberries in a high power food processor. Blend until smooth.

2. Add almond milk and blend again for twenty seconds.

3. Refrigerate the prepared smoothie for one hour.

4. Serve chilled.

Creamsicle Smoothie

Total Prep & Cooking Time: Ten minutes

Yields: Two servings

Nutrition Facts: Calories: 121.3 | Protein: 4.7g | Carbs: 19.8g | Fat: 2.5g | Fiber: 0.3g

Ingredients

- One cup of orange juice
- One and a half cup of crushed ice
- Half cup of milk
- One tsp. of white sugar

Method:

1. Blend milk, orange juice, white sugar, and ice in a high power blender.

2. Keep blending until there is no large chunk of ice. Try to keep the consistency of slushy.

3. Serve immediately.

Sunshine Smoothie

Total Prep & Cooking Time: Thirty minutes

Yields: Four servings

Nutrition Facts: Calories: 176.8 | Protein: 4.2g | Carbs: 39.9g | Fat: 1.3g | Fiber: 3.9g

Ingredients

- Two nectarines (pitted, quartered)
- One banana (cut in chunks)
- One orange (peeled, quartered)
- One cup of vanilla yogurt
- One-third cup of orange juice
- One tbsp. of honey

Method:

1. Add banana chunks, nectarines, and orange in a blender. Blender for two minutes.

2. Add vanilla yogurt, honey, and orange juice. Blend the ingredients until frothy and smooth.

3. Pour the smoothie in glasses and serve.

Chapter 3: Vegetable Smoothies

Apart from fruit smoothies, vegetable smoothies can also provide you with essential nutrients. In fact, vegetable smoothies are tasty as well. So, here are some vegetable smoothie recipes for you.

Mango Kale Berry Smoothie
Total Prep & Cooking Time: Ten minutes

Yields: Four servings

Nutrition Facts: Calories: 117.3 | Protein: 3.1g | Carbs: 22.6g | Fat: 3.6g | Fiber: 6.2g

Ingredients

- One cup of orange juice
- One-third cup of kale
- One and a half cup of mixed berries (frozen)
- Half cup of mango chunks
- One-fourth cup of water
- Two tbsps. of chia seeds

Method:

1. Take a high power blender and add kale, orange juice, berries, mango chunks, chia seeds, and half a cup of water.

2. Blend the ingredients on high settings until smooth.

3. In case the smoothie is very thick, you can adjust the consistency by adding more water.

4. Pour the smoothie in glasses and serve.

Breakfast Pink Smoothie

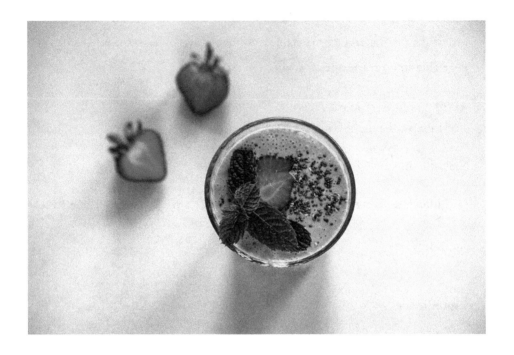

Total Prep & Cooking Time: Ten minutes

Yields: Two servings

Nutrition Facts: Calories: 198.3 | Protein: 12.3g | Carbs: 6.3g | Fat: 4.5g | Fiber: 8.8g

Ingredients

- One and a half cup of strawberries (frozen)
- One cup of raspberries
- One orange (peeled)

- Two carrots

- Two cups of coconut milk (light)

- One small beet (quartered)

Method:

1. Add strawberries, raspberries, and orange in a blender. Blend until frothy and smooth.

2. Add beet, carrots, and coconut milk.

3. Blend again for one minute.

4. Divide the smoothie in glasses and serve.

Butternut Squash Smoothie

Total Prep & Cooking Time: Five minutes

Yields: Four servings

Nutrition Facts: Calories: 127.3 | Protein: 2.3g | Carbs: 32.1g | Fat: 1.2g | Fiber: 0.6g

Ingredients

- Two cups of almond milk
- One-fourth cup of nut butter (of your choice)
- One cup of water
- One and a half cup of butternut squash (frozen)
- Two ripe bananas
- One tsp. of cinnamon (ground)
- Two tbsps. of hemp protein
- Half cup of strawberries
- One tbsp. of chia seeds
- Half tbsp. of bee pollen

Method:

1. Add butternut squash, bananas, strawberries, and almond milk in a blender. Blend until frothy and smooth.

2. Add water, nut butter, cinnamon, hemp protein, chia seeds, and bee pollen. Blend the ingredients f0r two minutes.

3. Divide the smoothie in glasses and enjoy!

Zucchini and Wild Blueberry Smoothie

Total Prep & Cooking Time: Ten minutes

Yields: Three servings

Nutrition Facts: Calories: 190.2 | Protein: 7.3g | Carbs: 27.6g | Fat: 8.1g | Fiber: 5.7g

Ingredients

- One banana
- One cup of wild blueberries (frozen)
- One-fourth cup of peas (frozen)
- Half cup of zucchini (frozen, chopped)
- One tbsp. of each
  - Hemp hearts
  - Chia seeds
  - Bee pollen
- One-third cup of almond milk
- Two tbsps. of nut butter (of your choice)
- Ten cubes of ice

Method:

1. Add blueberries, banana, peas, and zucchini in a high power blender. Blend the ingredients for two minutes.

2. Add chia seeds, hemp hearts, almond milk, bee pollen, nut butter, and ice. Blend the mixture for making a thick and smooth smoothie.

3. Pour the smoothie in glasses and serve with chopped blueberries from the top.

Cauliflower and Blueberry Smoothie

Total Prep & Cooking Time: Five minutes

Yields: Two servings

Nutrition Facts: Calories: 201.9 | Protein: 7.1g | Carbs: 32.9g | Fat: 10.3g | Fiber: 4.6g

Ingredients

- One Clementine (peeled)
- Three-fourth cup of cauliflower (frozen)
- Half cup of wild blueberries (frozen)
- One cup of Greek yogurt
- One tbsp. of peanut butter
- Bunch of spinach

Method:

1. Add cauliflower, Clementine, and blueberries in a blender. Blend for one minute.

2. Add peanut butter, spinach, and yogurt. Pulse the ingredients for two minutes until smooth.

3. Divide the prepared smoothie in glasses and enjoy!

Immunity Booster Smoothie

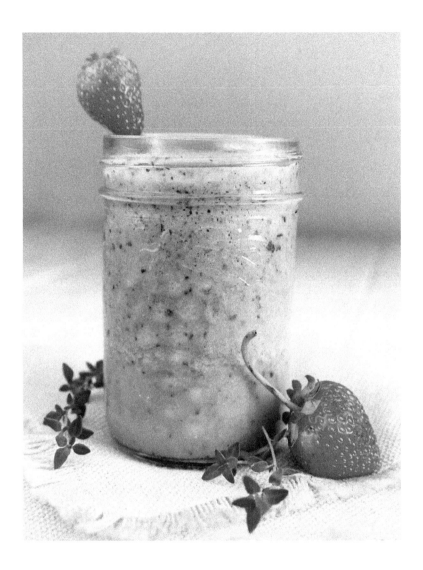

Total Prep & Cooking Time: Ten minutes

Yields: Two servings

Nutrition Facts: Calories: 301.9 | Protein: 5.4g | Carbs: 70.7g | Fat: 4.3g | Fiber:

8.9g

Ingredients

For the orange layer:

- One persimmon (quartered)
- One ripe mango (chopped)
- One lime (juiced)
- One tbsp. of nut butter (of your choice)
- Half tsp. of turmeric powder
- One pinch of cayenne pepper
- One cup of coconut milk

For the pink layer:

- One small beet (cubed)
- One cup of berries (frozen)
- One pink grapefruit (quartered)
- One-fourth cup of pomegranate juice
- Half cup of water
- Six leaves of mint
- One tsp. of honey

Method:

1. Add the ingredients for the orange layer in a blender. Blend for making a smooth liquid.

2. Pour the orange liquid evenly in serving glasses.

3. Add the pink layer ingredients in a blender. Blend for making a smooth liquid.

4. Pour the pink liquid slowly over the orange layer.

5. Pour in such a way so that both layers can be differentiated.

6. Serve immediately.

Ginger, Carrot, and Turmeric Smoothie

Total Prep & Cooking Time: Forty minutes

Yields: Two servings

Nutrition Facts: Calories: 140 | Protein: 2.6g | Carbs: 30.2g | Fat: 2.2g | Fiber: 5.6g

Ingredients

For carrot juice:

- Two cups of water
- Two and a half cups of carrots

For smoothie:

- One ripe banana (sliced)
- One cup of pineapple (frozen, cubed)
- Half tbsp. of ginger
- One-fourth tsp. of turmeric (ground)
- Half cup of carrot juice
- One tbsp. of lemon juice
- One-third cup of almond milk

Method:

1. Add water and carrots in a high power blender. Blend on high settings for making smooth juice.

2. Take a dish towel and strain the juice over a bowl. Squeeze the towel for taking out most of the juice.

3. Add the ingredients for the smoothie in a blender and blend until frothy and creamy.

4. Add carrot juice and blend again.

5. Pour the smoothie in glasses and serve.

Romaine Mango Smoothie

Total Prep & Cooking Time: Five minutes

Yields: Two servings

Nutrition Facts: Calories: 117.3 | Protein: 2.6g | Carbs: 30.2g | Fat: 0.9g | Fiber: 4.2g

Ingredients

- Sixteen ounces of coconut water
- Two mangoes (pitted)
- One head of romaine (chopped)
- One banana
- One orange (peeled)
- Two cups of ice

Method:

1. Add mango, romaine, orange, and banana in a high power blender. Blend the ingredients until frothy and smooth.

2. Add coconut water and ice cubes. Blend for one minute.

3. Pour the prepared smoothie in glasses and serve.

Fig Zucchini Smoothie

Total Prep & Cooking Time: Ten minutes

Yields: Two servings

Nutrition Facts: Calories: 243.3 | Protein: 14.4g | Carbs: 74.3g | Fat: 27.6g | Fiber: 9.3g

Ingredients

- Half cup of cashew nuts
- One tsp. of cinnamon (ground)
- Two figs (halved)
- One banana
- Half tsp. of ginger (minced)
- One-third tsp. of honey
- One-fourth cup of ice cubes
- One pinch of salt
- Two tsps. of vanilla extract
- Three-fourth cup of water
- One cup of zucchini (chopped)

Method:

1. Add all the listed ingredients in a high power blender. Blend for two minutes until creamy and smooth.

2. Pour the smoothie in serving glasses and serve.

Carrot Peach Smoothie

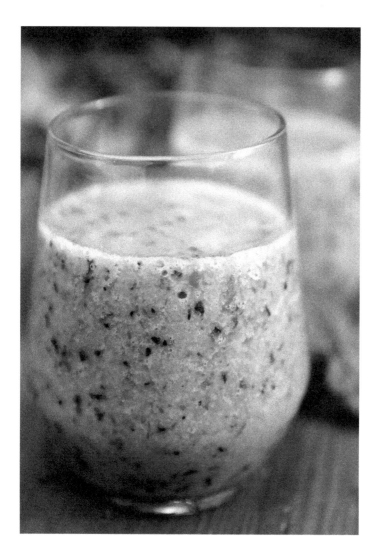

Total Prep & Cooking Time: Ten minutes

Yields: Two servings

Nutrition Facts: Calories: 191.2 | Protein: 11.2g | Carbs: 34.6g | Fat: 2.7g | Fiber: 5.4g

Ingredients

- Two cups of peach
- One cup of baby carrots
- One banana (frozen)
- Two tbsps. of Greek yogurt
- One and a half cup of coconut water
- One tbsp. of honey

Method:

1. Add peach, baby carrots, and banana in a high power blender. Blend on high settings for one minute.

2. Add Greek yogurt, honey, and coconut water. Give the mixture a whizz.

3. Pour the smoothie in glasses and serve.

Sweet Potato and Mango Smoothie

Total Prep & Cooking Time: Ten minutes

Yields: Two servings

Nutrition Facts: Calories: 133.3 | Protein: 3.6g | Carbs: 28.6g | Fat: 1.3g | Fiber: 6.2g

Ingredients

- One small sweet potato (cooked, smashed)
- Half cup of mango chunks (frozen)
- Two cups of coconut milk
- One tbsp. of chia seeds
- Two tsps. of maple syrup
- A handful of ice cubes

Method:

1. Add mango chunks and sweet potato in a high power blender. Blend until frothy and smooth.

2. Add chia seeds, coconut milk, ice cubes, and maple syrup. Blend again for one minute.

3. Divide the smoothie in glasses and serve.

Carrot Cake Smoothie

Total Prep & Cooking Time: Ten minutes

Yields: Two servings

Nutrition Facts: Calories: 289.3 | Protein: 3.6g | Carbs: 47.8g | Fat: 1.3g | Fiber: 0.6g

Ingredients

- One cup of carrots (chopped)
- One banana
- Half cup of almond milk
- One cup of Greek yogurt
- One tbsp. of maple syrup
- One tsp. of cinnamon (ground)
- One-fourth tsp. of nutmeg
- Half tsp. of ginger (ground)
- A handful of ice cubes

Method

1. Add banana, carrots, and almond milk in a blender. Blend until frothy and smooth.

2. Add yogurt, cinnamon, maple syrup, ginger, nutmeg, and ice cubes. Blend again for two minutes.

3. Divide the smoothie in serving glasses and serve.

Notes:

- You can add more ice cubes and turn the smoothie into slushy.

- You can store the leftover smoothie in the freezer for two days.

Chapter 4: Green Smoothies

Green smoothies can help in the process of detoxification as well as weight loss. Here are some easy-to-make green smoothie recipes for you.

Kale Avocado Smoothie

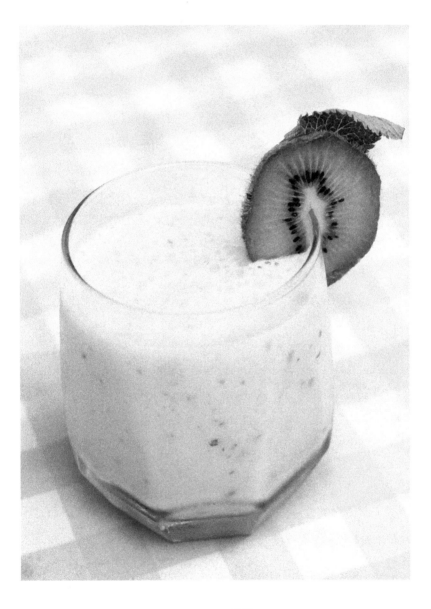

Total Prep & Cooking Time: Ten minutes

Yields: Two servings

Nutrition Facts: Calories: 401 | Protein: 11.2g | Carbs: 64.6g | Fat: 17.3g | Fiber: 10.2g

Ingredients

- One banana (cut in chunks)
- Half cup of blueberry yogurt
- One cup of kale (chopped)
- Half ripe avocado
- One-third cup of almond milk

Method:

1. Add blueberry, banana, avocado, and kale in a blender. Blend for making a smooth mixture.

2. Add the almond milk and blend again.

3. Divide the smoothie in glasses and serve.

Celery Pineapple Smoothie
Total Prep & Cooking Time: Ten minutes

Yields: Two servings

Nutrition Facts: Calories: 112 | Protein: 2.3g | Carbs: 3.6g | Fat: 1.2g | Fiber: 3.9g

Ingredients

- Three celery stalks (chopped)
- One cup of cubed pineapple
- One banana
- One pear
- Half cup of almond milk
- One tsp. of honey

Method:

1. Add celery stalks, pear, banana, and cubes of pineapple in a food processor. Blend until frothy and smooth.

2. Add honey and almond milk. Blend for two minutes.

3. Pour the smoothie in serving glasses and enjoy!

Cucumber Mango and Lime Smoothie

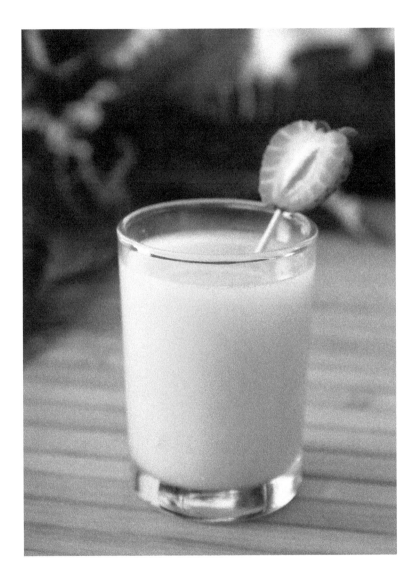

Total Prep & Cooking Time: Ten minutes

Yields: Two servings

Nutrition Facts: Calories: 165 | Protein: 2.2g | Carbs: 32.5g | Fat: 4.2g | Fiber: 3.7g

Ingredients

- One cup of ripe mango (frozen, cubed)
- Six cubes of ice
- Half cup of baby spinach leaves
- Two leaves of mint
- Two tsps. of lime juice
- Half cucumber (chopped)
- Three-fourth cup of coconut milk
- One-eighth tsp. of cayenne pepper

Method:

1. Add mango cubes, spinach leaves, and cucumber in a high power blender. Blend until frothy and smooth.

2. Add mint leaves, lime juice, coconut milk, cayenne pepper, and ice cubes. Process the ingredients until smooth.

3. Pour the smoothie in glasses and serve.

Kale, Melon, and Broccoli Smoothie

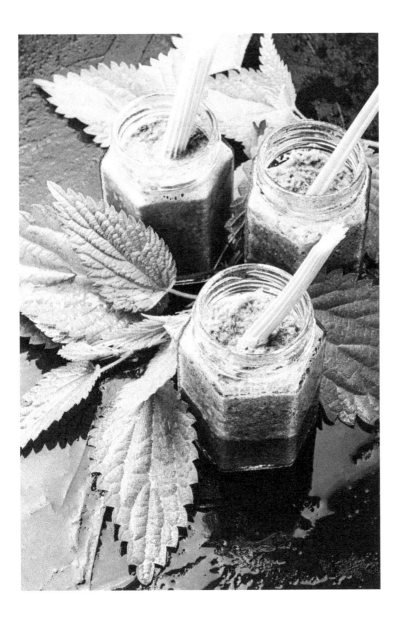

Total Prep & Cooking Time: Ten minutes

Yields: One serving

Nutrition Facts: Calories: 96.3 | Protein: 2.3g | Carbs: 24.3g | Fat: 1.2g | Fiber: 2.6g

Ingredients

- Eight ounces of honeydew melon
- One handful of kale
- Two ounces of broccoli florets
- One cup of coconut water
- Two sprigs of mint
- Two dates
- Half cup of lime juice
- Eight cubes of ice

Method:

1. Add kale, melon, and broccoli in a food processor. Whizz the ingredients for blending.

2. Add mint leaves and coconut water. Blend again.

3. Add lime juice, dates, and ice cubes. Blend the ingredients until smooth and creamy.

4. Pour the smoothie in a smoothie glass. Enjoy!

Kiwi Spinach Smoothie

Total Prep & Cooking Time: Ten minutes

Yields: Two servings

Nutrition Facts: Calories: 102 | Protein: 3.6g | Carbs: 21.3g | Fat: 2.2g | Fiber: 3.1g

Ingredients

- One kiwi (cut in chunks)
- One banana (cut in chunks)
- One cup of spinach leaves
- Three-fourth cup of almond milk
- One tbsp. of chia seeds
- Four cubes of ice

Method:

1. Add banana, kiwi, and spinach leaves in a blender. Blend the ingredients until smooth.

2. Add chia seeds, ice cubes, and almond milk. Blend again for one minute.

3. Pour the smoothie in serving glasses and serve.

Avocado Smoothie

Total Prep & Cooking Time: Ten minutes

Yields: Two servings

Nutrition Facts: Calories: 345 | Protein: 9.1g | Carbs: 47.8g | Fat: 16.9g | Fiber: 6.7g

Ingredients

- One ripe avocado (halved, pitted)
- One cup of milk
- Half cup of vanilla yogurt
- Eight cubes of ice
- Three tbsps. of honey

Method:

1. Add avocado, vanilla yogurt, and milk in a blender. Blend the ingredients until frothy and smooth.

2. Add honey and ice cubes. Blend the ingredients for making a smooth mixture.

3. Serve immediately.

PART III

Chapter 1: Identifying the Mediterranean Diet

We know that certain diets are associated with better health—this is a simple fact of life. We've seen that entire groups of people live longer based on where they live, and to some degree, a good deal of that has to come from somewhere—it has to come from something like diet or environment. In this case, the diet of the people living in the Mediterranean has been found to be incredibly healthy for people—it has been shown that people who are able to enjoy this diet, who are able to eat fresh food by the sea and enjoy the benefits that it has, are able to be far healthier than those who don't have it. That is great for them—but what is their secret?

It turns out, it's all in the lifestyle. The Mediterranean lifestyle, food, and all, is incredibly healthy for you. Studies have shown that people living in Mediterranean countries such as Greece and Italy have been found to have far less risk of death from coronary disease. Their secret is in the diet. Their diet has been shown to reduce the risk of cardiovascular disease, meaning that it is incredibly healthy, beneficial, and something that the vast majority of people in the world could definitely benefit from.

The Mediterranean diet is recommended by doctors and the World Health Organization as being not only healthy but also sustainable, meaning that it is something that is highly recommended, even by the experts. If you've found that you've struggled with weight loss, heart disease, managing your blood pressure, or anything similar to those problems, then the Mediterranean diet is for you. When you follow this diet, you are able to bring health back to your life and enjoy the foods while doing so. It's perfect if you want to be able to enjoy your diet without having to worry about the impacts that it will have on you.

Defining the Mediterranean Lifestyle

The Mediterranean diet is quite simple. It involves eating traditional foods based on one's location. Typically, in the Mediterranean, that is a diet that is rich in veggies, fruits, whole grains, beans, and features olive oil as the fat of choice. Typically, it involves elements beyond just eating as well. While it is important to have healthy food, it is equally important to recognize that the diet encompasses the lifestyle as well. In particular, you can expect to see a few other rules come into play.

In particular, the Mediterranean diet is unique in the sense that it encourages a glass of red wine every now and then. In fact, the diet is associated with moderate drinking, enjoying red wine several times per week, always responsibly, and in contexts that will be beneficial to the drinker. If you want to be able to enjoy the Mediterranean diet and you are pregnant, or against drinking, you can do that, too—but traditionally, the red wine is included and even encouraged in moderation thanks to the antioxidants within it.

Additionally, on the Mediterranean diet, it is common to share meals with friends and family. This is essential—eating is more than just filling the body, it is nurturing the mind and relationships as well. This also comes with the added benefit of also being able to slow down eating—when you are eating the foods on this diet, you will discover that ultimately, you eat less when you're busy having a riveting conversation with someone. The fact that you are slowed down with your eating means that you will fill up sooner and realize that you didn't have to actually eat the food that you did. This means that you eat less and are, therefore managing your portions better as a result.

Finally, the Mediterranean diet focuses on physical activity. Traditionally, you would have had to go out to get the foods that you would eat each day, and that would mean that you'd need to get up, fish, garden, farm, or otherwise prepare your food. Eating locally is still a major component of this diet, as is getting up and being active. You need at least 30 minutes of activity, moderate or mild, per day. Even just walking for half an hour is better than nothing!

The Rules of the Mediterranean Diet

To eat the Mediterranean way, there are a few key factors that can guide you. If you know what you are doing, you can eat well without having to sacrifice flavor for health, and that matters immensely. When you look at the Mediterranean diet closely, you see that there are several tips that will help you to recognize what you need to do to stick to your diet.

Eating fruits and veggies

First, make sure that the bulk of your calories come from fruits and vegetables. You should be eating between 7 and 10 servings of fresh fruits and vegetables every single day—meaning that the bulk of your calories will come from there. Try to stick to locally grown foods that are fresh and in-season—they will have the highest nutritional value.

Reach for the whole grains

Yes, pasta is a major part of the diet in the Mediterranean, and you don't have to give that up entirely—but make sure that any grains that you are enjoying are whole-wheat. This allows you to enjoy foods that are high in fiber and are able to be digested differently than when you use refined carbs instead. While the refined carbs may give you instantaneous energy, they are also not nearly as good for you as whole wheat.

Using healthy fats

When it comes to flavoring or cooking your foods, you need to reach for the healthy fats first. This means choosing out foods that are cooked with olive oil instead of butter or dipping food in olive oil instead of butter. Olive oil, despite being a fat, has not been found to lead to weight gain when used in moderation. It is an incredibly healthy substitute for butter that is loaded up with all sorts of beneficial, heart-healthy antioxidants that will help your cardiovascular system.

Aim for seafood

When it comes to protein, fish, especially fresh fish, is the best choice. Fish should be consumed at least twice per week, and it should be fresh rather than frozen whenever possible. In particular, it is commonly recommended that you reach for salmon or trout, or other fatty fish because the omega-3 fatty acids within them are incredibly healthy for you, and they will serve you well. Even better, if you grill your fish, you have little cleanup.

Reduce red meat

In addition to adding more seafood to your diet, you need to cut out the red meat. The red meats in your diet are no good for you—they have been linked to inflammation that can make it harder for your cardiovascular system.

Enjoy dairy in moderation

When you are on this diet, dairy is not out of the picture entirely. While you should avoid butter, for the most part, it is a good idea for you to enjoy some low-fat Greek yogurt on occasion and add in some cheese to your diet. It is a good thing for you to enjoy these foods to ensure that you have plenty of calcium to keep your body strong.

Spices, not salt

Perhaps one of the most profound differences between most other diets and the Mediterranean diet is the lack of salt. The Mediterranean diet reaches for herbs and spices before adding in salt, meaning that you will be consuming less of it over time. Even better, you will grow to love your new foods without needing salt.

Chapter 2: Savory Mediterranean Meals

Mediterranean Feta Mac and Cheese

Ingredients

- Egg (1, beaten)
- Feta cheese (8 oz., crumbles)
- Macaroni (0.5 lb., whole-wheat)
- Olive oil (3 Tbsp.)
- Salt and pepper to taste
- Sour cream (8 oz.)

Instructions

1. Cook pasta to instructions to create al dente pasta. Drain and place pasta into baking dish. Toss in feta and oil and mix well.
2. Combine your egg and sour cream with salt and pepper. Then mix well and toss over macaroni. Combine and bake at 350F for 30 minutes.

Chickpea Stew

Ingredients

- Bay leaf (1)
- Dry chickpeas (1 c., soaked overnight and peeled)
- Garlic (1 clove, cut in half)
- Lemon to serve

- Olive oil (0.25 c.)
- Onion (1, diced)
- Salt and pepper to taste

Instructions

1. Cover chickpeas in pot with just enough water to cover them and wait to boil. Then rinse and set into clean pot. Toss in all other ingredients but the lemon with just enough water to cover nearly one inch above the beans. Simmer for 2-3 hours and serve with lemons.

Savory Mediterranean Breakfast Muffins

Ingredients

Dry ingredients

- Baking powder (1.5 tsp)
- Baking soda (o.5 tsp)
- Flour (2 c.)
- Salt (0.5 tsp)

Wet ingredients

- Egg (1 large)
- Garlic (1 clove, minced)
- Milk (1 c.)
- Sour cream (0.25 c.)
- Vegetable oil (0.25 c.)

Fillings

- Cheddar cheese (2 c., shredded)
- Feta (2.5 oz., crumbled)
- Green olives (diced, 0.5 c.)
- Green onions (0.5 c., chopped)
- Roasted red peppers (0.5 c., chopped)
- Sun dried tomatoes (diced, 0.5 c.)

Instructions

1. Combine dry ingredients in a bowl. Mix wet ingredients in separate bowl. Combine the two together and mix.
2. Toss in fillings in as few stirs as possible.
3. Place in greased or lined muffin pan, dividing to all 12 recesses.
4. Bake for 25 minutes until golden-brown and crusty at 350F.
5. Cool for 10 minutes and serve warm.

Mediterranean Breakfast Bake

Ingredients

- Artichoke hearts (14-oz. can, drained)
- Bread (6 slices whole-wheat, chopped)
- Eggs (8)
- Feta cheese (0.5 c.)
- Italian sausage (turkey or chicken—1 lb., casings removed)
- Milk (1 c.)
- Olive oil (2 Tbsp., divided)

- Onion (1, chopped)
- Spinach (5 oz.)
- Sun dried tomato (1 c., chopped)

Instructions

1. Warm 1 Tbsp. of your olive oil on moderately high heat. Cook sausage for 8 minutes until it has browned, breaking it up as it cooks. Place it in a dish when it is done.
2. Toss in additional oil, then cook onion until soft, roughly 5 minutes. Toss in spinach until wilting (1 minute).
3. Combine eggs and mix in milk, bread, tomatoes, cheese, artichokes, sausage, and finally, the spinach mix.
4. Place everything in a 2.5 quart baking dish. Let sit for an hour in fridge, or leave overnight.
5. Let casserole sit for 30 minutes after removing from fridge. Then, bake for 45 minutes at 350F until brown. Let rest 10 minutes, then serve.

Mediterranean Pastry Pinwheels

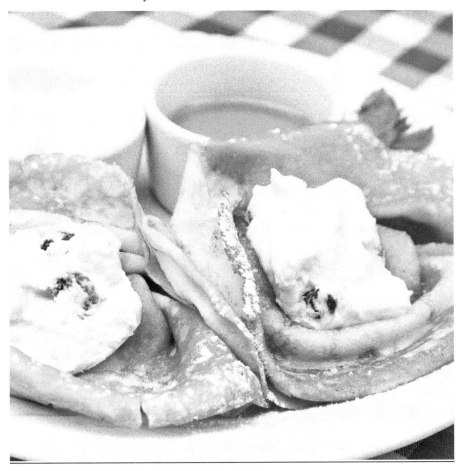

Ingredients

- Cream cheese (8-ounce package, softened)
- Pesto (0.25 c.)
- Provolone cheese (0.75 c.)
- Sun-dried tomatoes (0.5 c., chopped)
- Ripe olives (0.5 c., chopped)

Instructions

1. Unroll pastry and trim it up to create 10-inch square.
2. Mix together your cream cheese and pesto until well-combined. Then, mix in other ingredients until combined. Place mixture in even layer across pastry, up to 0.5-inch of edges. Roll and freeze for 30 minutes.
3. Cut whole roll into 16 pieces.
4. Bake at 400F until golden, roughly 15 minutes. Serve.

Chapter 3: Sweet Treats on the Mediterranean Diet

Greek Yogurt Parfait

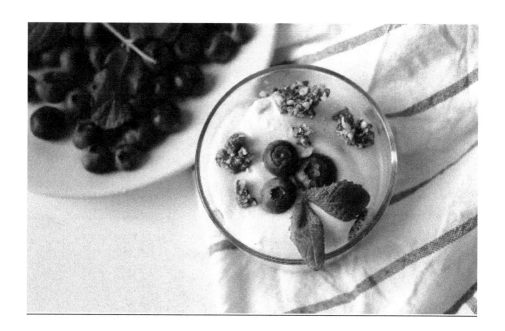

Ingredients

- Almond butter (2 Tbsp.)
- Fresh fruit (1 Tbsp.)
- Greek Yogurt (1 c.)

Instructions

1. Mix together yogurt and 1 Tbsp. of almond butter and put in a bowl. Top with fruit.

2. Warm remaining butter in microwave for 10 minutes, then drizzle atop yogurt. Serve. You can add different toppings to change up the flavor as well.

Overnight Oats

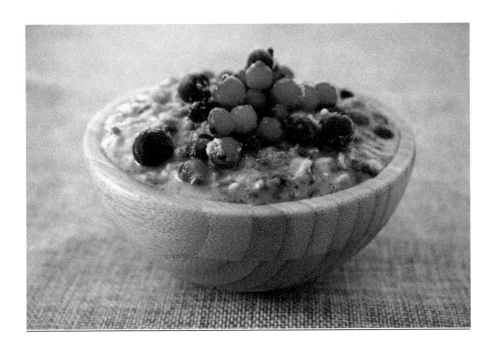

Ingredients

- Chia seeds (1 Tbsp.)
- Greek yogurt (0.25 c.)
- Honey (1 Tbsp.)
- Milk of choice (0.5 c.)
- Old fashioned whole oats (0.5 c.)
- Vanilla extract (0.25 tsp)

Instructions

1. Mix all ingredients into a glass container and leave in fridge for at least 2 hours but preferably overnight. Serve with berries of choice or other desired toppings.

Apple Whipped Yogurt

Ingredients

- Greek yogurt (1 c.)
- Heavy cream (0.5 c.)
- Honey (1 Tbsp.)
- Unsalted butter (2 Tbsp.)
- Apples (2, cored and chopped into small bits)
- Sugar (2 Tbsp.)
- Cinnamon (1/8 tsp)
- Walnut halves (0.25 c., chopped)

Instructions

1. Using a hand mixer, mix together yogurt, honey, and honey until it creates peaks.
2. Heat up your butter in a skillet over a moderate temperature. Cook apples and 1 Tbsp. sugar in pan. Stir and cook for 6-8 minutes until soft. Then, top with the rest of sugar and cinnamon, stirring and cooking an additional 3 minutes. Take it off of the burner and let it rest for 5 minutes.
3. Serve with whipped yogurt in bowl topped with apple, then sprinkle on walnuts.

Chapter 4: Gourmet Meals on the Mediterranean Diet

Garlic-Roasted Salmon and Brussels Sprouts

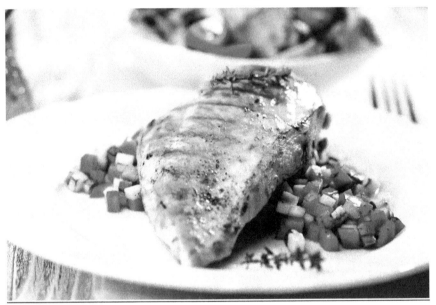

Ingredients

- Brussels sprouts (6 c., trimmed and halved)
- Chardonnay (0.75 c.)
- Garlic cloves (14 large)
- Olive oil (0.25 c.)
- Oregano (2 Tbsp., fresh)
- Pepper (0.75 tsp)
- Salmon fillet (2 lbs., skin-off—cut in 6 pieces)
- Salt (1 tsp)

- Lemon wedges to serve

Instructions

1. Take two cloves of garlic and mince, combining them with oil, 1 Tbsp. of oregano, half of the salt and 1/3 of the pepper. Cut remaining cloves of garlic in halves and toss them with the sprouts. Take 3 Tbsp. of your garlic oil and toss it with the sprouts in roasting pan. Roast for 15 minutes at 450F.

2. Add wine to the remainder of the oil mixture. Then, remove it from the pan, stir veggies, and place salmon atop it all. Pour the wine mix atop it and season with remaining oregano and salt and pepper. Bake 5-10 minutes until salmon is done. Serve alongside the wedged lemon.

Walnut Crusted Salmon with Rosemary

Ingredients

- Dijon mustard (2 tsp)
- Garlic (1 clove, minced)
- Honey (0.5 tsp)
- Kosher salt (0.5 tsp)
- Lemon juice (1 tsp)
- Lemon zest (0.25 tsp.)
- Olive oil (1 tsp)
- Olive oil spray
- Panko (3 Tbsp.)
- Red pepper (0.25 tsp)

- Rosemary (1 tsp, chopped)
- Salmon (1 pound, skin removed)
- Walnuts (3 Tbsp., finely chopped)
- Parsley and lemon to garnish

Instructions

1. Mix together the mustard, lemon zest and juice, honey, salt and red pepper, and rosemary. In a separate dish, combine the panko with oil and walnuts.
2. Spread mustard across salmon and top with panko mixture. Spray fillets with cooking spray.
3. Cook until fish begins to flake at 425F, roughly 8-10 minutes. Serve with lemon and parsley.

Spaghetti and Clams

Ingredients

- Clams (6.5 lbs.)
- Olive oil (6 Tbsp.)
- White wine (0.5 c.)
- Garlic (3 cloves, sliced)
- Chiles (3, small and crumbled)
- Spaghetti (1 lb.)
- Parsley (3 Tbsp., chopped)
- Salt and pepper to personal preference

Instructions

1. Prepare clams, soaking in clean water and brushing to remove all sand.

2. Warm 2 Tbsp. of oil in large pot. Then, toss in 0.25 c. wine, 1 of the cloves of garlic, and 1 chile. Cook half of the plans at high heat with regular shaking until clams are opened. Remove opened clams and their juices to a larger bowl. Repeat process with second half of clams. Discard any that do not open.

3. Prepare pasta according to packaging to create al dente pasta. Reserve 1 c. pasta water.

4. Warm remainder of oil (2 Tbsp.) in pot over moderate heat, tossing in remainder of garlic and chile. Cook until fragrant, then place all clams and their juices into the pot, tossing to coat well. Then, toss in pasta, mixing well to combine. If necessary, add in cooking liquid. Serve and season with salt/pepper to personal preference with parsley atop.

Braised Lamb and Fennel

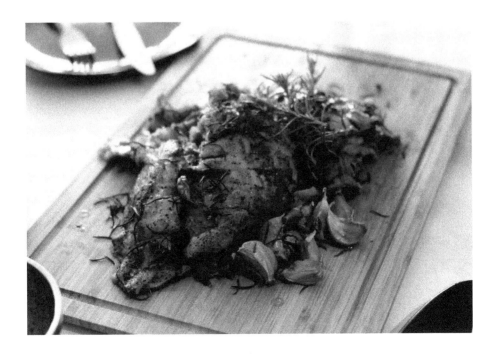

Ingredients

- Bay leaves (2)
- Chicken broth (3 c.)
- Cinnamon stick (1)
- Fennel (1 bulb, chopped)
- Garlic head (chopped in half)
- Lamb shoulder (3 lbs., cut into 8 pieces)
- Olive oil (2 Tbsp.)
- Onion (1, chopped
- Orange (1 with peel, cut into wedges)
- White wine (1 c.)
- Whole peeled tomatoes (14.5 oz. can)

Instructions

1. Dry lamb and season with salt and pepper to taste. Warm oil inside a Dutch oven, and sear lamb on all sides, roughly 6 minutes each side. Move lamb to plate.

2. Place fennel, garlic, and onion in the pot and cook, until browning, roughly 8 minutes. Mix in wine and boil, deglazing the pan. Reduce heat and simmer until it has reduced 50%.

3. Toss in orange, bay leaves, tomatoes, broth, and cinnamon, plus the lamb. Simmer, then cover pot and transfer to oven set to 325F. braise for 1.5-2 hours. Remove lamb and place on clean plate.

4. Strain liquid left in pot, then return it to the pot to boil until thick, roughly 30 minutes.

5. Return lamb to pot to warm. Serve.

Mediterranean Cod

Ingredients

- Black olives (0.66 c., sliced)
- Cod (4 fillets, skinless)
- Fennel seeds (1 tsp)
- Lemon (1, sliced)
- Lemon (juice of ½ lemon)
- Olive oil (6 Tbsp.)
- Onion (1, sliced)
- Parsley (1 Tbsp., chopped)
- Salt and pepper to personal preference
- Tomatoes (0.66 c., diced)

Instructions

1. Warm olive oil at a moderate temperature, sautéing the onion with a pinch of salt until translucent, roughly 10 minutes.
2. Mix in tomato and olives, tossing in the juice as well. Allow it to simmer gently for roughly 5 minutes. Toss in fennel seeds and set aside.
3. Warm the rest of the oil in another pan and fry up the cod for 10 minutes, flipping halfway through until done.
4. Toss tomato sauce over heat to warm, then mix together the parsley, and serve atop the cod with a lemon slice.

Baked Feta with Olive Tapenade

Ingredients

- Baked pita or crusty bread to serve
- Feta cheese (6 oz.)
- Garlic (2 cloves)
- Green olives (0.33 c., sliced)
- Harissa paste (3 Tbsp.)
- Olive oil (3 Tbsp.)
- Parsley (3 Tbsp., fresh chopped)
- Roasted red peppers (16-oz. jar, drained)
- Salt (0.75 tsp.)
- Tomato paste (2 Tbsp.)
- Walnuts (0.5 c., halved)

Instructions

1. In a blender, combine your peppers, 0.25 c. walnuts, harissa and tomato paste, garlic, and 0.5 tsp of your salt until mostly consistent. It doesn't have to be perfect, but should be well combined.
2. Take half of mixture into baking dish that has been sprayed with cooking spray. Top with half of your feta, then spoon the rest of the red pepper sauce atop it.
3. Top with the last of the feta and bake until bubbly, roughly 25 minutes. Broil for the last 2.
4. While that bakes, make your tapenade. This requires you to combine your remaining ingredients together.
5. Remove mixture from oven and top with tapenade. Serve immediately with crusty bread or pita chips.

Chapter 5: 30-Minutes or Less Meals

Vegetarian Toss Together Mediterranean Pasta Salad

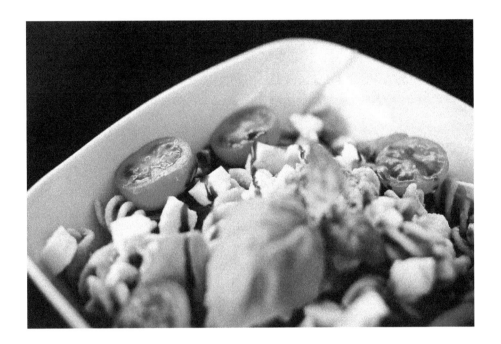

Ingredients

- Artichoke hearts (12 oz. jar, drained)
- Balsamic vinegar (2 Tbsp.)
- Kalamata olives (12-ounce jar, drained and chopped)
- Olive oil (2 Tbsp.)
- Pasta (8 oz., wheat)
- Salt to personal preference

- Sun-dried tomatoes in oil (1.5 oz. jar, drained)

Instructions

1. Prepare pasta according to packaging.
2. Mix together olives, tomatoes, and artichoke.
3. Drain pasta and add them to a bowl with artichoke mixture. Then, top with vinegar and olive oil, mix well, and serve warm.

Vegetarian Aglio e Olio and Broccoli

Ingredients

- Olive oil (3 Tbsp.)
- Cayenne peppers (3)
- Garlic (3 cloves, sliced)
- Broccoli (1 head, prepared in florets)
- Spaghetti (7 oz. whole wheat)
- Salt to taste

Instructions

1. Boil water and prepare spaghetti according to instructions until al dente. Drain and reserve.
2. In a pan, heat up 1 Tbsp. of your olive oil at a moderate temperature, then toss in the garlic and peppers, sautéing until fragrant. Remove garlic from heat and set aside.
3. Toss broccoli into pan and cook for 4 minutes. Then toss in spaghetti, garlic, and remaining oil. Cook for an additional minute or two, then serve.

Cilantro and Garlic Baked Salmon

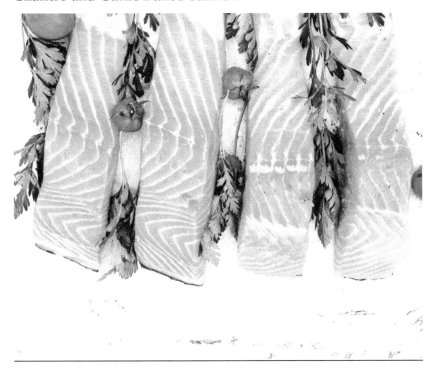

Ingredients

- Cilantro (stems trimmed)

- Garlic (4 cloves, chopped)

- Lime (0.5, cut into rounds)

- Lime juice (1 lime's worth)

- Olive oil (0.5 c.)

- Salmon fillet (2 pounds, skin removed)

- Salt to taste

- Tomato (cut into rounds)

Instructions

1. Allow salmon to come to room temp for 20 minutes while oven preheats to a temperature of 425 F.

2. While you wait, take a processor and combine garlic, cilantro, lime juice, and olive oil with a pinch of salt. Combine well.

3. Place fillet into baking pan that has been greased. Top with a light sprinkle of salt and pepper. Then spread cilantro sauce atop fillet, coating whole salmon. Top with tomato and lime.

4. Bake for 6 minutes per 0.5 inch of thickness (1-inch fillets take around 8-10 minutes). Let rest for 5-10 minutes out of the oven. Serve.

Harissa Pasta

Ingredients

- Pasta (2 cups)
- Red bell pepper (1)
- Red onion (1)
- Pine nuts (2 Tbsp.)
- Harissa paste (2 Tbsp.)

Instructions

1. Roast onions and peppers with olive oil at 400F for 20 minutes. Remove from oven and dice.

2. Prepare pasta to instructions on package. While pasta cooks, toast your pine nuts until browned in frying pan.

3. Drain pasta, leaving a touch of the water. Then, add in diced roasted veggies and harissa. Serve topped with pine nuts.

Chapter 6: 1-Hour-or-Less Meals

1 Hour Baked Cod

Ingredients

- Basil (0.5 tsp., dried)
- Bay leaf (1)
- Capers (1 small jar)
- Cod fillets (2 pounds)
- Fennel seeds (1 tsp., crushed)
- Garlic (1 clove, minced)
- Lemon juice (0.25 c., fresh)
- Olive oil (2 tsp)
- Onion (1, sliced)
- Orange juice (o.25 c., fresh)
- Orange peel (1 Tbsp.)
- Oregano (0.5 tsp., dried)
- Salt and pepper to personal preference
- White wine (1 c., dry)
- Whole tomatoes (16-oz. can, chopped and reserving juice)

Instructions

1. Warm oven to 375F.

2. In cast iron skillet, warm oil. Then, sauté your onion for 5 minutes. At this point, mix in all other ingredients but fish. Allow to simmer for 30 minutes.

3. Place fillets into skillet and top with most of the sauce. Allow to bake for 15 minutes until fish flakes.

Grilled Chicken Mediterranean Salad

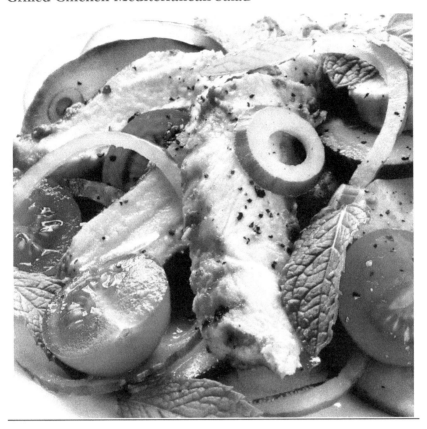

Ingredients

- Artichoke hearts (0.33 c., chopped)
- Balsamic vinegar (2 Tbsp.)
- Basil (1 tsp, dried)
- Chicken breasts (3, cut into bite-sized chunks)
- Cucumber (0.75 c., diced)
- Feta cheese (0.25 c.)
- Garlic (1 clove, minced)
- Greek yogurt (2 Tbsp.)
- Green onions (0.25 c., chopped)
- Kalamata olives (3 Tbsp., sliced)

- Kosher salt (0.5 tsp)
- Lemon juice (3 Tbsp + 1 tsp.)
- Olive oil (3 Tbsp. + 2 Tbsp.)
- Onion powder (0.5 tsp)
- Parsley (0.5 tsp)
- Pesto (4 tsp)
- Pinch of red pepper
- Roasted red pepper (6 Tbsp., sliced)
- Romaine (4 c., chopped)
- Shiitake mushrooms
- Spinach (4 c., chopped)
- Tomato (0.75 c., diced)
- White wine vinegar (4 tsp)

Instructions

1. Create your salad. Each plate should have a bed of romaine and spinach, topped with cucumber, tomato, artichoke, peppers, olives, and cheese.

2. Combine your tsp of lemon juice, wine vinegar, and pesto in a jar and shake to combine. Then, add in yogurt and 2 Tbsp. oil, mixing well until well-incorporated.

3. Prepare your chicken. Let it marinade in a mixture of 3 Tbsp. lemon juice, balsamic vinegar, remaining oil, and all seasonings for at least 30 minutes. Soak some wooden skewers in water during this time.

4. Make kebabs out of chicken and mushroom, alternating bite of chicken and bite of mushroom until chicken is gone. Grill for 10 to 15 minutes until done.

5. Drizzle salad with the vinaigrette, then place a kebab atop each. Serve.

Lemon Herb Chicken and Potatoes One Pot Meal

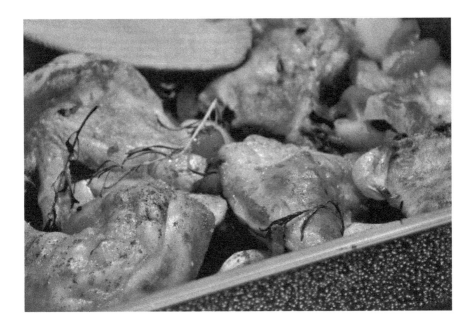

Ingredients

- Baby potatoes (8, halved)
- Basil (3 tsp, dried)
- Bell pepper (1, seeds removed and wedged)
- Chicken thighs (4, skin and bone on)
- Garlic (4 large cloves, crushed)
- Kalamata olives (4 Tbsp., pitted)
- Lemon juice (1 lemon's worth)
- Olive oil (3 Tbsp.)
- Oregano (2 tsp, dried)
- Parsley (2 tsp, dried)

- Red onion (wedged)
- Red wine vinegar (1 Tbsp.)
- Salt (2 tsp)
- Zucchini (1 large, sliced)
- Lemons for garnish

Instructions

1. Combine juice from lemon, 2 Tbsp. olive oil, vinegar, seasonings, and garlic into dish. Pour half to reserve for later, then place chicken in half. Let sit for 15 minutes (or overnight if you would like to prep the day before)

2. Warm oven to 430F. Sear chicken in cast iron skillet in remaining olive oil, about 4 minutes per side. Drain all but 1 Tbsp. of fat.

3. Place all veggies around the thighs. Top with remaining marinade and combine well to cover everything.

4. Cover pan and bake for 35 minutes until soft and chicken is to temperature. Then, broil for 5 minutes or until golden brown. Top with olives and lemon to serve.

Vegetarian Mediterranean Quiche

Ingredients

- Butter (2 Tbsp.)
- Cheddar cheese (1 c., shredded)
- Eggs (4 large)
- Feta (0.33 c.)
- Garlic (2 cloves, minced)
- Kalamata olives (0.25 c., sliced)
- Milk (1.25 c.)
- Onion (1, diced)
- Oregano (1 tsp, dried)
- Parsley (1 tsp, dried)
- Pie crust (1, prepared)
- Red pepper (1, diced)
- Salt and pepper to personal preference
- Spinach (2 c., fresh)
- Sun dried tomatoes (0.5 c.)

Instructions

1. Soak sun-dried tomatoes in boiling water for 5 minutes before draining and chopping.
2. Prepare a pie dish with a crust, fluting the edges.
3. In a skillet, melt your butter, then cook your garlic and onions in it until they become fragrant. Combine in the red peppers for another 3 minutes until softened. Then, toss in your spinach, olives, and seasoning. Cook

until the spinach wilts, about 5 minutes. Take it off of the heat and toss in your feta and tomatoes. Then, carefully place mixture into the crust, spreading it into a nice, even layer.

4. Mix milk, eggs, and half of cheddar cheese together. Pour it into the crust. Then, top with cheddar.

5. Bake for 50 minutes at 375 f. until crust is browned and egg is done.

Herbed Lamb and Veggies

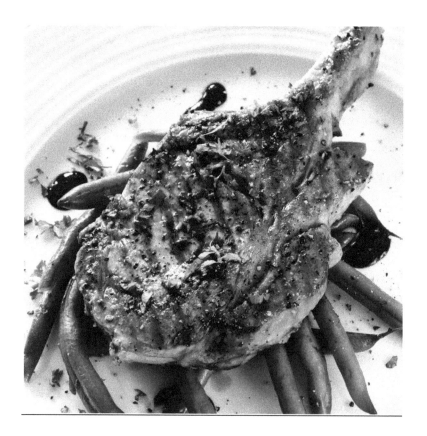

Ingredients

- Bell pepper (2, any color, seeds removed and cut into bite-sized chunks)
- Lamb cutlets (8 lean)
- Mint (2 Tbsp., fresh, chopped)
- Olive oil (1 Tbsp.)
- Red onion (1, wedged)
- Sweet potato (1 large, peeled, and chunked)
- Thyme (1 Tbsp., fresh, chopped)
- Zucchini (2, chunked)

Instructions

1. Assemble your veggies onto a baking sheet and coat with oil and black pepper. Bake at 400F for 25 minutes.
2. As veggies bake, trim fat from the lamb. Then, combine the herbs with a bit of freshly ground pepper. Coat the lamb in the seasoning.
3. Remove veggies, flip, and push to one side of pan. Then, arrange your cutlets onto the baking pan as well. Bake for 10 minutes, flip, then cook an additional 10 minutes. Combine well, then serve.

Chicken and Couscous Mediterranean Wraps

Ingredients

- Parsley (1 c., fresh and chopped)
- Olive oil (3 Tbsp.)

- Garlic (2 tsp, minced)
- Salt (pinch)
- Pepper (pinch)
- Chicken tenders (1 pound)
- Tomato (1, chopped)
- Cucumber (1, chopped)
- Spinach wraps (4 1o-inch)
- Water (0.5 c)
- Mint (0.5 c., fresh chopped)
- Lemon juice (0.25 c.)
- Couscous (0.33 c.)

Instructions

1. Cook couscous in boiling water according to directions on package.
2. Mix together your lemon juice, oil, garlic, salt and pepper, mint, and parsley.
3. Coat chicken in 1 Tbsp. of your mixture from previous step and top with a pinch of salt. Cook in skillet until completely cooked, usually just a few minutes per side.
4. Wait for chicken to cool, then chop into bites.
5. Pour the remainder of your parsley mixture into the couscous with cucumbers and tomato bits.
6. Place 0.75 c. of couscous mixture into a tortilla, then spread chicken atop it, rolling them up and serving.

Sheet Pan Shrimp

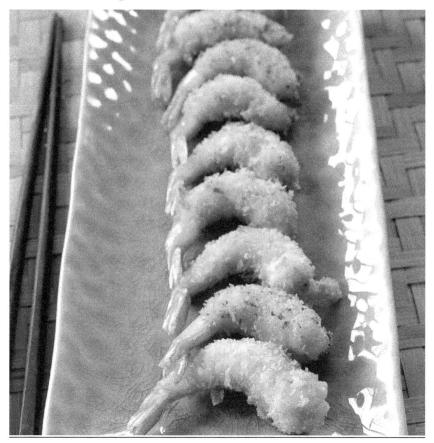

Ingredients

For shrimp

- Feta cheese (0.5 c.)

- Fingerling potatoes (2 c., halved)

- Green beans (6 oz., trimmed)

- Olive oil (3 Tbsp.)
- Pepper (1 tsp)
- Red onion (1 medium, sliced)
- Red pepper (1 medium, sliced)
- Salt (1 tsp)
- Shrimp (1 lb., deveined and peeled)

For Marinade

- Garlic (1 Tbsp., minced)
  Oregano (0.5 tsp)
- Greek yogurt (1 c.)
- Lemon juice (2 Tbsp.)
- Paprika (0.5 tsp)
- Parsley (2 Tbsp., chopped)

Instructions

1. Combine all marinade ingredients and set aside.
2. Take shrimp in a bowl with 0.5 c. of the marinade. Let them sit for 30 minutes.
3. During rest time, set up your baking sheet with foil or parchment, and prepare your veggies. Chop them up and toss onto baking sheet, drizzling them with the olive oil and giving them a quick sprinkle of salt and pepper. Bake for roughly 20 minutes at 400F, then remove from oven. Take out all green beans and set to the side.
4. Place shrimp in one layer across the pan and bake for an additional 10 minutes until shrimp is done. Serve with veggies and shrimp in bowls, topped with 2 Tbsp. feta and a spoonful of yogurt marinade.

Mediterranean Mahi Mahi

Ingredients

- Basil (6 leaves, freshly chopped)
- Capers (4 Tbsp.)
- Garlic (2 cloves, chopped)
- Italian seasoning (pinch)
- Kalamata olives (25, chopped)
- Lemon juice (1 tsp)
- Mahi mahi (1 pound)
- Olive oil (2 Tbsp.)
- Onion (0.5, chopped)
- Parmesan cheese (3 Tbsp.)
- Diced tomatoes (15 oz. can)
- White wine (0.25 c.)

Instructions

1. Warm olive oil in a pan and then cook onions until translucent. Toss in garlic and seasoning and stir to mix well. Then, add in your can of tomatoes, wine, olives, lemon, and roughly half of the chopped basil. Drop heat down and toss in parmesan cheese. Cook until bubbling.
2. Put fish into a baking pan, then top with the sauce. Bake for 20 minutes at 425 F until fish is to temperature.

Chapter 7: Slow Cooker Meals

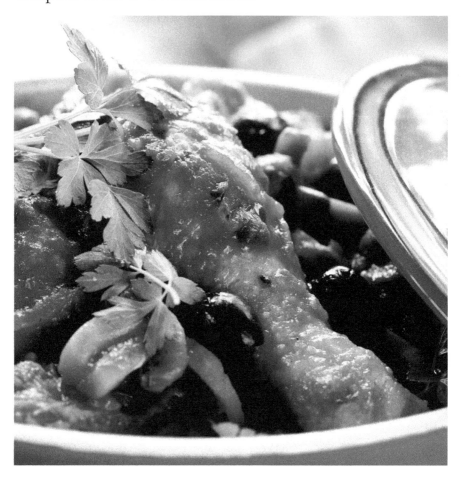

Slow Cooker Mediterranean Chicken

Ingredients

- Bay leaf (1)
- Capers (1 Tbsp.)
- Chicken broth (0.5 c.)
- Chicken thighs (2 pounds, bone and skin removed)

- Garlic (3 cloves, minced)
- Kalamata olives (1 c.)
- Olive oil (1 Tbsp.)
- Oregano (1 tsp)
- Roasted red pepper (1 c.)
- Rosemary (1 tsp, dried)
- Salt and pepper to taste
- Sweet onion (1, thinly sliced)
- Thyme (1 tsp, dried)
- Optional fresh lemon wedges to juice for serving

Instructions

1. Sauté the chicken in olive oil to brown on both sides, then remove it from the pan. Then, sauté the onions and garlic as well until beginning to soften, roughly 5 minutes.
2. Put chicken, onion, garlic, and all other ingredients into a slow cooker and leave it to cook for 4 hours on low. Season to taste.

Slow Cooker Vegetarian Mediterranean Stew

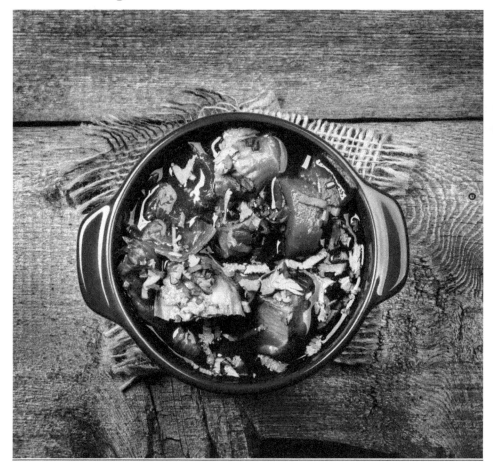

Ingredients

- Carrot (0.75 c., chopped)

- Chickpeas (15 oz. can)

- Crushed red pepper (0.5 tsp)

- Fire-roasted diced tomatoes (2 14-oz. cans)

- Garlic (4 cloves, minced)

- Ground pepper (0.25 tsp)

- Kale (8 c., chopped)

- Lemon juice (1 Tbsp.)
- Olive oil (3 Tbsp.)
- Onion (1, chopped)
- Oregano (1 tsp)
- Salt (0.75 tsp)
- Vegetable broth (3 c.)
- Basil leaves (garnish)
- Lemon wedges (garnish)

Instructions

1. Mix tomatoes, onion, carrot, broth, seasonings, and garlic into the slow cooker. Cook on low for 6 hours.
2. Take out 0.25 c. of the liquid in the slow cooker after 6 hours and transfer it to a bowl. Take out 2 Tbsp. of chickpeas and mash them with the liquid until nice and smooth.
3. Combine mash, kale, juice from lemon, and whole chickpeas. Cook for about 30 minutes, until kale is tender, then serve garnished with the basil leaves and lemon wedges.

Vegetarian Slow Cooker Quinoa

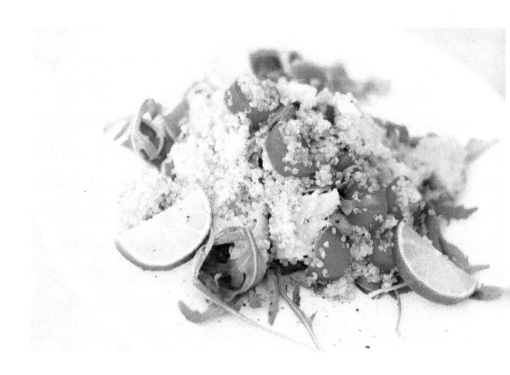

Ingredients

- Arugula (4 c.)
- Chickpeas (1 15.5 oz. can, rinsed and drained)
- Feta cheese (0.5 c)
- Garlic (2 cloves, minced)
- Kalamata olives (12, halved)
- Kosher salt (0.75 tsp)
- Lemon juice (2 tsp)

- Olive oil (2.25 Tbsp.)

- Oregano (2 Tbsp., fresh and coarsely chopped

- Quinoa (1.5 c., uncooked)

- Red onion (1 c., sliced)

- Roasted red pepper (0.5 c., drained and chopped)

- Vegetable stock (2.25 c.)

Instructions

1. Mix your broth with the onion, garlic, quinoa, chickpeas, and 1.5 tsp of olive oil. Sprinkle half of the salt atop it. Mix and cook on low until quinoa is done, roughly 3 or 4 hours.

2. Turn off the slow cooker and mix well. In a separate bowl, combine remaining olive oil, salt, and lemon juice together. Then, mix that into the slow cooker, along with the peppers.

3. Combine in the arugula and leave until the greens start to wilt. Serve, topping with feta, oregano, and olives.

Slow-Cooked Chicken and Chickpea Soup

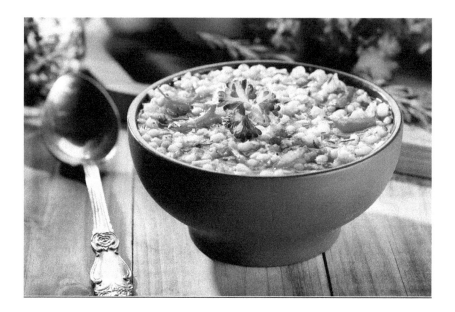

Ingredients

- Artichoke hearts (14 oz. can, drained and chopped)
- Bay leaf (1)
- Cayenne (0.25 tsp)
- Chicken thighs (2 lbs., skins removed)
- Cumin (4 tsp)
- Diced tomatoes (1 15-ounce can)
- Dried chickpeas (1.5 c., allow to soak overnight)
- Garlic cloves (4, chopped)
- Olives (o.25 c., halved)
- Paprika (4 tsp)
- Pepper (0.25 tsp)

- Salt (0.5 tsp)
- Tomato paste (2 Tbsp.)
- Water (4 c.)
- Yellow onion (chopped)
- Parsley or cilantro (garnish)

Instructions

1. Drain your soaked chickpeas and place them into your slow cooker (large preferred). Mix in the water, onions and garlic, tomatoes (undrained), tomato paste, and all seasonings. Combine well, then add in the chicken.

2. Leave it to cook for 8 hours at low, or 4 at high.

3. Remove the chicken and allow it to cool on a cutting board. At the same time, remove the bay leaf, then add in the artichoke and olives. Season with additional salt if necessary to taste. Chop up chicken, removing the bones, and then mix it back into the soup. Serve the soup with the parsley or cilantro garnishing the top.

Slow Cooked Brisket

Ingredients

- Beef broth (0.5 c.)
- Brisket (3 lbs.)
- Cold water (0.25 c.)
- Fennel bulbs (2, cored, trimmed, and cut into wedges)
- Flour
- Italian seasoning (3 tsp)
- Italian seasoning diced tomatoes (14.5 oz. can)
- Lemon peel (1 tsp., fine shreds)
- Olives (0.5 c.)
- Parsley for garnish
- Pepper (pinch)
- Salt (pinch)

Instructions

1. Trim meat, then season with 1 tsp Italian seasoning. Put it in slow cooker with the cut-up fennel on top.
2. Mix together the tomatoes, broth, peel, olives, salt and pepper, and the last of the Italian seasoning.
3. Cook at low for 10 hours, or high for 5.
4. Take meat out of the cooker and reserve all juice. Arrange meat with veggies on a serving platter.
5. Remove fat from top of the juices.
6. Take 2 c. of juices in saucepan. Mix together water and flour, then combine it into the juice. Cook until gravy forms.
7. Serve meat topped with gravy and garnish with parsley.

Vegan Bean Soup with Spinach

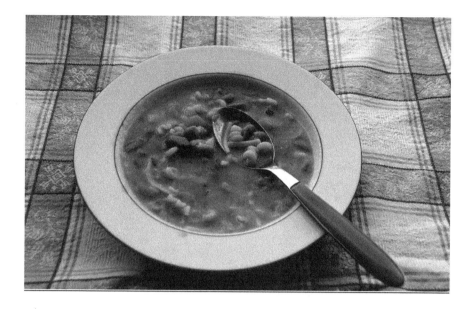

Ingredients

- Vegetable broth (3 14-oz. cans)
- Tomato puree (15 oz. can)
- Great Northern or White beans (15 oz. can)
- White rice (0.5 c)
- Onion (0.5 c., chopped)
- Garlic (2 cloves, minced)
- Basil (1 tsp., dried)
- Pinch of salt
- Pinch of pepper
- Kale or spinach (8 c., chopped)

Instructions

1. Mix everything but leafy greens together in your slow cooker. Cook for 5 or 7 hours on low, or 2.5 hours on high.

2. Toss in leafy greens. Wait for them to wilt and serve.

Moroccan Lentil Soup

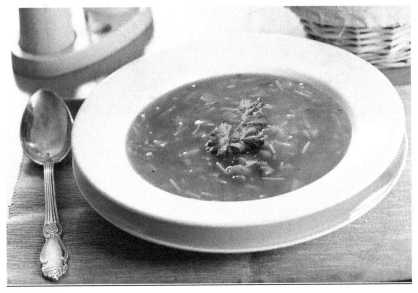

Ingredients

- Carrots (2 c., chopped)
- Cauliflower (3 c.)
- Cinnamon (0.25 tsp)
- Cumin (1 tsp)
- Diced tomato (28 oz.)

- Fresh cilantro (0.5 c.)
- Fresh spinach (4 c.)
- Garlic (4 cloves, minced)
- Ground coriander (1 tsp)
- Lemon juice (2 Tbsp.)
- Lentils (1.75 c.)
- Olive oil (2 tsp)
- Onion (2 c., chopped)
- Pepper (pinch)
- Tomato paste (2 Tbsp.)
- Turmeric (1 tsp)
- Vegetable broth (6 c.)
- Water (2 c.)

Instructions

1. Mix everything but spinach, cilantro, and lemon juice. Cook until lentils soften. This will be 4-5 hours if you use high heat, or 10 hours on low.
2. Mix spinach when just 30 minutes remains on cook time.
3. Just before serving, top with cilantro and lemon juice.

Chapter 8: Vegetarian and Vegan Meals

Vegetarian Greek Stuffed Mushrooms

Ingredients

- Cherry tomatoes (0.5 c., quartered)
- Feta cheese (0.33 c.)
- Garlic (1 clove, mixed)
- Ground pepper (0.5 tsp)
- Kalamata olives (2 Tbsp.)
- Olive oil (3 Tbsp.)
- Oregano (1 Tbsp., fresh and roughly chopped)
- Portobello mushrooms (4, cleaned with stems and gills taken out)
- Salt (0.25 tsp)
- Spinach (1 c., chopped)

Instructions

1. Begin by setting your oven. This recipe requires 400F for baking.
2. Mix together your salt and 0.25 tsp pepper, garlic, and 2 Tbsp. of oil, and use it to cover your mushrooms, inside and out.
3. Set the mushrooms onto your baking pan and allow it to cook for 10 minutes.

4. Mix together your remaining ingredients and combine well. Then, when the mushrooms are done, remove them from the oven and then fill them up with your filling.

5. Allow to cook for another 10 minutes.

Vegetarian Cheesy Artichoke and Spinach Stuffed Squash

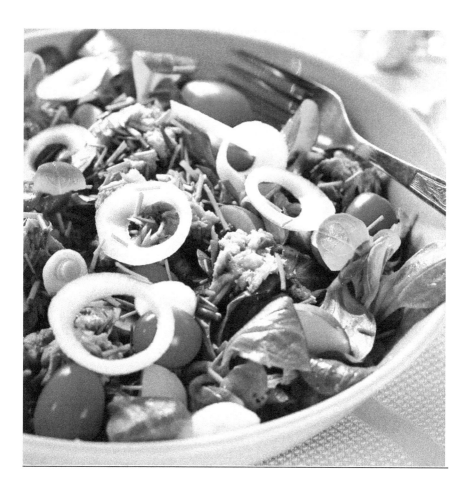

Ingredients

- Artichoke Hearts (10 oz., frozen—thawed and chopped up)
- Baby spinach (5 oz.)
- Cream cheese (4 oz., softened)
- Parmesan cheese (0.5 c.)
- Pepper (pinch to taste)
- Red pepper and basil (for garnish)
- Salt (pinch to taste)
- Spaghetti squash (1, cut in half and cleaned out of seeds)
- Water (3 Tbsp.)

Instructions

1. Microwave your squash, flat side down, with 2 Tbsp. of your water uncovered for 10-15 minutes.
2. Mix together your spinach and water into a skillet until they begin to wilt. Then drain and reserve for later.
3. Preheat your oven set to broil with the rack at the upper 1/3 point.
4. Remove flesh from squash with a fork, then place the shells onto a sheet for the oven. Then stir in your artichoke, cheeses, and a pinch of salt and pepper to the squash flesh. Combine thoroughly, then split it between the two shells. Broil for 3 minutes and top with red pepper and basil to taste.

Vegan Mediterranean Buddha Bowl

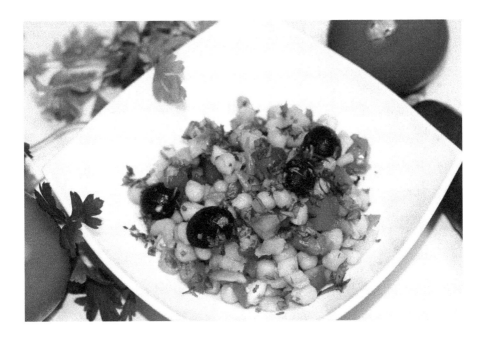

Ingredients

For the chickpeas

- Chickpeas (1 can, rinsed, drained, and skinned)
- Olive oil (1 tsp)
- Pinch of salt and pepper
- Dried basil (0.25 tsp)
- Garlic powder (0.25 tsp)

For the quinoa

- Quinoa (0.5 c.)
- Water (1 c.)

For the salad

- Bell pepper (1, color of choice, seeded, stemmed, and chopped to bite-sized bits)
- Cucumbers (2, peeled and chopped)
- Grape tomatoes (1 c., halved)
- Hummus (0.5 c.)
- Kalamata olives (0.5 c.)
- Lettuce (2 c. – can sub in field greens, spinach, kale, or any other leafy greens)

Instructions

1. Set your oven up to prepare for baking. It should be at 0400F. Then, mix the ingredients for the chickpeas together, coating them evenly with the seasoning.
2. Put chickpeas in single layer and put them onto the baking sheet. Roast for 30 minutes with an occasional mixing and rotation of the pan to allow them all to cook evenly. Allow them to cool.
3. Start preparing the quinoa and water in a microwave-safe bowl. Combine the water and quinoa and microwave, covered, for 4 minutes. Then stir and microwave for 2 minutes longer. Give it one final stir and leave it to rest in the microwave for another minute or two.
4. Begin assembling your salad. Begin with the greens at the bottom, then top with tomatoes, cucumbers, bell pepper, olives, chickpeas, and then quinoa. Finally, top with a dollop of hummus to serve.

Vegan Mediterranean Pasta

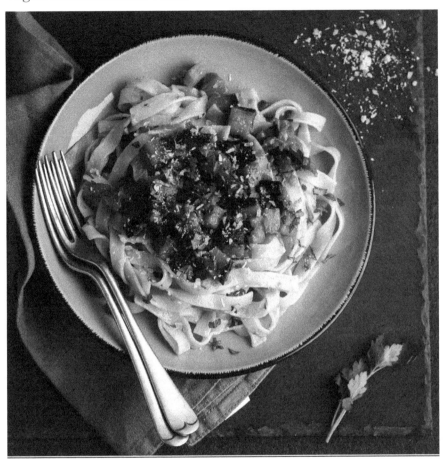

Ingredients

- Artichokes (0.5 c.)
- Basil leaves (0.25 c., torn)
- Garlic cloves (2-3 to taste, minced)
- Grape tomatoes (2 c., halved)
- Kalamata olives (10, pitted)
- Olive oil (1 Tbsp.)
- Pasta (8 oz.)

- Red pepper (0.25 tsp.)
- Salt and pepper to taste
- Spinach (4 c.)
- Tomato paste (4 Tbsp.)
- Vegetable broth (1 c.)

Instructions

1. Prepare your pasta based on the instructions provided. Keep 1 c. of the water for later use and then set the pasta aside.
2. While preparing your pasta, take the time to warm a large skillet with oil. Then, sauté your garlic and red pepper for 30 seconds or so. Combine in the tomato paste and cook for another minute. At that point, mix in your tomatoes, your seasoning, your artichokes and olives, and your broth. Let it cook until tomatoes start to break down.
3. Mix in the pasta to the tomato mixture. Let it cook another 2 minutes and add reserved pasta water if too dry.
4. Add in spinach and basil and cook until wilted.
5. Remove from heat and serve.

Vegetarian Zucchini Lasagna Rolls

Ingredients

- Basil (2 Tbsp., fresh)
- Egg (1, lightly beaten)
- Frozen spinach (10-ounce package, thawed and dried)
- Garlic (1 clove)
- Marinara sauce (0.75 c.)
- Olive oil (2 tsp)
- Parmesan cheese (3 Tbsp.)
- Pinch each of salt and pepper
- Ricotta (1.33 c.)
- Shredded mozzarella cheese (8 Tbsp.)
- Zucchini (2, trimmed)

Instructions

1. Prepare two baking sheets with cooking spray. Then set the oven to 425F.
2. Cut up your zucchini into strips lengthwise into 1/8 inch thick pieces. A mandolin will make this easier.
3. Prepare zucchini coated in oil with salt and pepper, then set up a flat layer across the bottom of the prepared pan.
4. Bake zucchini for 10 minutes until it begins to soften.
5. Mix together 2 Tbsp. mozzarella and 1 Tbsp. of parmesan. Then, in another bowl, combine egg, ricotta, spinach, garlic, and the remainder of the cheese. Toss in a pinch of salt and pepper and mix well.

6. Set up an 8-inch square casserole dish with 0.25 c. marinara spread across the bottom.

7. Take your zucchini that has been softened and begin to roll it. To do this, you will need to put 1 Tbsp. of ricotta mix at the bottom of your strip, then roll. Put the seam down in the marinara-covered bottom. Do this for all pieces of zucchini.

8. Cover the rolls with the remainder of your marinara sauce and top with the cheese mix.

9. Bake until bubbling, roughly 20 minutes. Rest for 5 minutes and top with basil.

Vegetarian Breakfast Sandwich

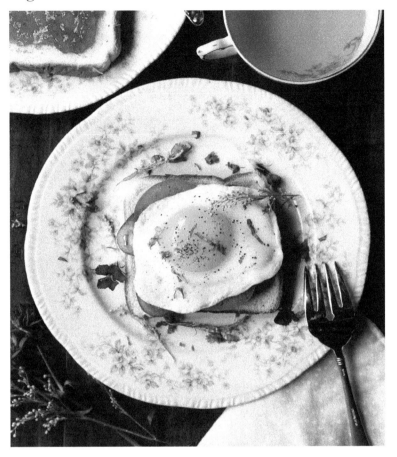

Ingredients

- Sandwich thins (2)
- Olive oil (2 Tbsp. + 1 tsp)
- Rosemary (1 Tbsp. fresh, or 0.5 tsp dried)
- Eggs (2)
- Spinach leaves (1 c.)
- Tomato (0.5, sliced thinly)
- Feta (2 Tbsp.)

- Pinch of salt and pepper

Instructions

1. Warm oven to 375F. Separate your sandwich thins and coat with olive oil. Bake for 5 minutes until beginning to crisp up.
2. Warm skillet with last tsp of olive oil. Break eggs into pan and cook until whites are set. Then, break the yolks and flip to finish cooking.
3. Put bottoms of the bread onto serving plates. Then, top with spinach, the tomato, one egg each, followed by the feta. Sprinkle with salt and pepper, then top with remaining bread.

Vegan Breakfast Toast

Ingredients

- Bread of choice (verify that it is vegan—2 slices)
- Spice blend of choice
- Arugula (handful)
- Tomato (1, cut into rounds)
- Chopped olives (1 Tbsp.)
- Cucumber (0.5, cut into rounds)
- Hummus (0.25 c.)

Instructions

1. Toast up your bread. Then spread the hummus across, season it, and top with all toppings split between the pieces.

Vegetarian Shakshouka

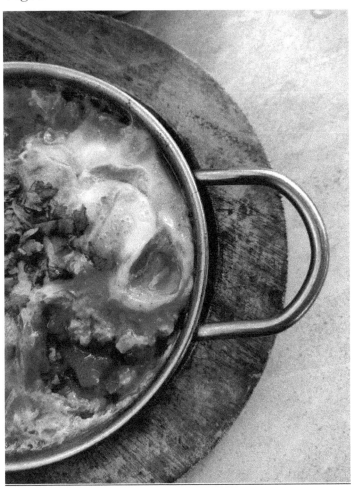

Ingredients

- Chopped parsley (1 Tbsp.)
- Diced Tomatoes (15 oz. can)
- Eggs (4)
- Garlic (2 cloves)

- Olive oil (2 Tbsp.)
- Onion (1—sliced)
- Red bell peppers (2, sliced thinly)
- Salt and pepper to taste
- Spicy harissa (1 tsp)
- Sugar (1 tsp)

Instructions

1. Warm oil in a cast iron pan. Sauté your peppers and onions until they have begun to soften, giving them a stir every now and then to prevent sticking. Add in the garlic for another minute.
2. Put in tomatoes, sugar, and harissa, leaving it to simmer for the next 7 minutes.
3. Season it to taste. Then, add in small indentations into the mixture in the pan, cracking an egg in each indentation that you make. Cover up the pot and allow it to cook until egg whites are done.

Cover with parsley and serve with bread.

PART IV

Vegetarian Cookbook

The vegetarian diet has gained immense popularity in the last few years. According to some studies, it has been found that an estimated 18% of the world population is vegetarian. Apart from all the environmental and ethical benefits of removing meat from the diet, a properly planned vegetarian diet can reduce the risk of various chronic diseases, improve diet quality, and help in losing weight. The vegetarian diet also does not include poultry and fish. The majority of the people opt for a vegetarian diet for personal or religious reasons and for ethical reasons, such as animal rights. Other people opt for it for various environmental reasons, like livestock production, which results in the emission of greenhouse gases.

A vegetarian diet comes along with a wide array of benefits. It has been found that vegetarians have a better quality of diet when compared to meat-eaters. They also have a higher intake of beneficial nutrients, such as vitamin C, fiber, magnesium, and vitamin E. Switching from a normal meat diet to a vegetarian diet can result to be an effective strategy in case you want to lose weight. For instance, in a review of twelve studies, it has been found that vegetarians can lose about four pounds of weight over eighteen weeks than non-vegetarians. Also, vegetarians have lower BMI or body mass index than non-vegetarians.

Some research found that a vegetarian diet can be linked to a lower risk of developing cancer and those of the colon, breast, stomach, and rectum. However, it lacks enough evidence to prove that a vegetarian diet can effectively reduce cancer risk. People who follow a vegetarian diet can maintain healthy levels of blood sugar. It can also help in preventing the onset of diabetes by controlling the levels of blood sugar. Vegetarian diets help in the reduction of various heart diseases that can make your heart stronger and healthier.

A vegetarian diet needs to include a wide mixture of veggies, fruits, healthy fats, grains, and proteins. To replace the protein that you get from meat in a diet, you will need to include plant foods rich in proteins such as seeds, nuts, legumes, seitan, tofu, and tempeh. Consuming whole foods rich in nutrients, such as vegetables and fruits, can provide your body with the necessary minerals and vitamins to fill the nutritional gaps in a diet. Some of the food items that you can include in your diet are:

- **Fruits:** Bananas, apples, melons, oranges, peaches, pears

- **Vegetables:** Asparagus, leafy greens, carrots, broccoli

- **Legumes:** Beans, lentils, chickpeas, peas

- **Seeds:** Chia, flaxseed, hemp

- **Nuts:** Walnuts, cashews, almonds

- **Proteins:** Seitan, natto, tofu, eggs, tempeh

You cannot include food items such as fish, seafood, meat, poultry, and ingredients that are based on meat. Restriction of eggs and dairy products are applicable for the vegans and not for vegetarians. I have included some tasty and easy vegetarian recipes that will help you to plan your diet effectively.

Chapter 1: Breakfast Recipes

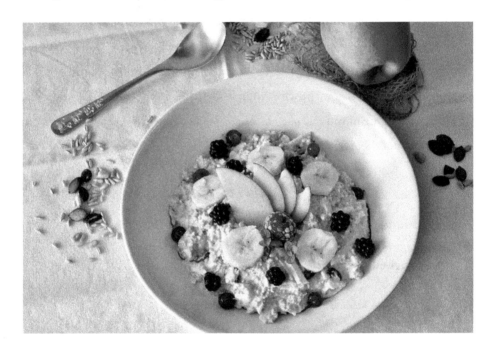

No matter which diet you follow, breakfast is very important in all cases. In this section, you will find some easy-to-make and tasty breakfast recipes that you can include in your vegetarian diet.

Black Bean Bowl

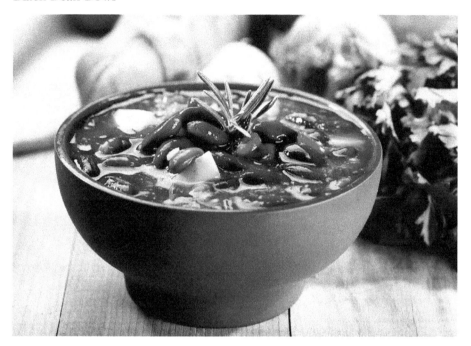

Total Prep & Cooking Time: Fifteen minutes

Yields: Two servings

Nutrition Facts: Calories: 620.1 | Protein: 28.9g | Carbs: 47.6g | Fat: 37.1g | Fiber: 23.2g

Ingredients:

- Two tbsps. of olive oil
- Four eggs (beaten)

- One can of black beans (rinsed)

- One avocado (sliced)

- One-fourth cup of salsa

- One tsp. of each

    o   Black pepper (ground)

    o   Salt

Method:

1. Take a small pan and heat oil in it. Add the eggs and scramble for five minutes.

2. Place the beans in a bowl. Heat the beans in the oven for one minute.

3. Divide the beans into two serving bowls.

4. Top the beans with scrambled eggs, salsa, and avocado. Add pepper and salt according to taste.

Coconut Blueberry Ricotta Bowl

Total Prep & Cooking Time: Twenty minutes

Yields: One serving

Nutrition Facts: Calories: 303.2 | Protein: 9.5g | Carbs: 32.1g | Fat: 15.3g | Fiber: 3.9g

Ingredients:

- One-fourth cup of ricotta cheese
- One tbsp. of each
    - Honey
    - Coconut milk
    - Slivered almonds
    - Coconut flakes
- Half cup of blueberries

Method:

1. Combine coconut milk and ricotta in a medium-sized bowl. Drizzle honey from the top and add coconut and almonds.

2. Serve with blueberries from the top.

Broccoli Quiche

Total Prep & Cooking Time: Fifty minutes

Yields: Six servings

Nutrition Facts: Calories: 378.2 | Protein: 17.3g | Carbs: 21.1g | Fat: 25.8g | Fiber: 3.1g

Ingredients:

- One pie crust (unbaked)
- Three tbsps. of butter
- One onion (minced)
- One tsp. of each
  - Garlic (minced)
  - Salt
- Two cups of broccoli (chopped)
- One and a half cup of mozzarella cheese (shredded)
- Four eggs (beaten)
- Two and a half cup of milk
- Half tsp. of black pepper
- One tbsp. of butter (melted)

Method:

1. Start by preheating your oven at 175 degrees Celsius. Use pie crust for lining a deep pie pan.

2. Take a large saucepan and add butter to it. Add broccoli, onion, and garlic. Cook the veggies slowly until tender. Add the cooked veggies to the pie crust and add cheese from the top.

3. Mix milk and eggs in a bowl; add pepper and salt for seasoning. Add the remaining butter to the milk mixture. Pour the mixture over the mixture of vegetables.

4. Bake the quiche in the oven for forty minutes or until the center has properly set.

Tomato Bagel Sandwich

Total Prep & Cooking Time: Twenty minutes

Yields: One serving

Nutrition Facts: Calories: 346.3 | Protein: 13.1g | Carbs: 48.6g | Fat: 10.7g | Fiber: 2.9g

Ingredients:

- One bagel (split, toasted)
- Two tbsps. of cream cheese
- One large tomato (sliced thinly)
- Pepper and salt (to season)
- Four basil leaves

Method:

1. Spread the cream cheese on the halves of the bagel.

2. Top the cheese layer with slices of tomato. Add pepper and salt for seasoning.

3. Serve with basil leaves from the top.

Cornmeal And Blueberry Pancakes

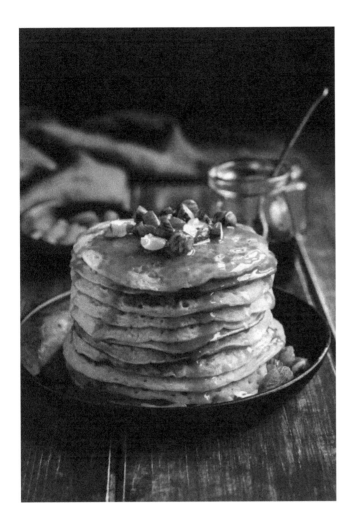

Total Prep & Cooking Time: Thirty minutes

Yields: Six servings

Nutrition Facts: Calories: 180.3 | Protein: 5.2g | Carbs: 26.8g | Fat: 5.1g | Fiber: 4.6g

Ingredients:

- One cup of soy milk
- Half cup of each
  - Water
  - Cornmeal (ground)
- One and a half cup of wheat flour
- One tsp. baking powder
- One-third tsp. baking soda
- One-fourth tsp. of salt
- One cup of blueberries
- Two tbsps. of vegetable oil

Method:

1. Preheat your oven at 95 degrees Celsius.

2. Combine water and soy milk in a bowl.

3. Take a large mixing bowl and combine cornmeal, baking soda, flour, salt, and baking powder. Add the mixture of soy milk. Combine properly. Add the blueberries and allow the batter to rest for five minutes.

4. Take a large skillet and grease it using oil. Add one-fourth cup of the batter in the skillet. Cook until the pancakes are bubbly on the top, and the edges are dry. Cook for five minutes on each side. Repeat with the remaining batter.

5. Serve hot with jam or syrup.

Breakfast Tortilla

Total Prep & Cooking Time: Twenty minutes

Yields: Two servings

Nutrition Facts: Calories: 381.3 | Protein: 15.8g | Carbs: 38.1g | Fat: 18.7g | Fiber: 4.5g

Ingredients:

- Two tbsps. of beans (refried)
- Three tbsps. of salsa
- Three large eggs (beaten)
- One tbsp. of mayonnaise
- Four tortillas (flour)
- One and a half cup of lettuce (shredded)

Method:

1. Combine salsa and beans in a small bowl.

2. Take an iron skillet and heat oil in it. Add the eggs and let the bottom set—Cook for one minute. Spread the mixture of beans on half of the egg and flip one side for making the shape of a half-circle. Cook until the eggs set properly.

3. Spread mayonnaise on the tortillas.

4. Cut the cooked eggs into four equal pieces. Place each piece of eggs on the tortillas. Top with lettuce.

5. Roll the tortillas. Serve hot.

Zucchini Frittata
Total Prep & Cooking Time: Forty minutes

Yields: Five servings

Nutrition Facts: Calories: 258.3 | Protein: 14.2g | Carbs: 9.1g | Fat: 19.6g | Fiber: 3.4g

Ingredients:

- One cup of water
- Three tbsps. of olive oil
- Half tsp. of salt
- Half bell pepper (green, chopped)
- Three zucchinis (cut in slices of half-inch)
- Two garlic cloves (peeled)
- One onion (diced)
- Six mushrooms (chopped)
- One tbsp. of butter
- Five eggs
- Pepper and salt (to taste)
- One and a half cup of mozzarella cheese (shredded)
- Three tbsps. of parmesan cheese

Method:

1. Start by preheating your oven at 160/175 degrees Celsius.

2. Take a large skillet and combine olive oil, water, green pepper, salt, garlic cloves, and zucchini. Simmer the mixture until the zucchini is soft— Cook for seven minutes.

3. Drain the water and remove the garlic; add mushroom, onion, and butter. Keep cooking until the onion turns transparent. Add the eggs and keep stirring. Add pepper and salt for seasoning. Cook until the eggs are firm.

4. Add mozzarella cheese from the top.

5. Bake in the oven for ten minutes.

6. Remove the frittata from the oven and add parmesan cheese from the top. Place under the broiler for about five minutes.

7. Cut the frittata in wedges and serve warm.

Oatmeal And Strawberry Smoothie

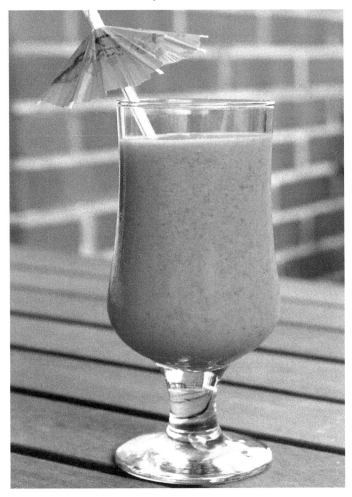

Total Prep & Cooking Time: Twenty minutes

Yields: Two servings

Nutrition Facts: Calories: 204.1 | Protein: 5.2g | Carbs: 41.3g | Fat: 2.7g | Fiber: 6.9g

Ingredients:

- One cup of almond milk
- Half cup of rolled oats
- Fourteen strawberries (frozen)
- One banana (cut in chunks)
- Two tsps. of agave nectar
- Half tsp. of vanilla extract

Method:

1. Add almond milk, strawberries, oats, agave nectar, banana, and vanilla extract in a food processor. Keep blending until smooth.

2. Serve with pieces of strawberry from the top.

Chapter 2: Appetizers Recipes

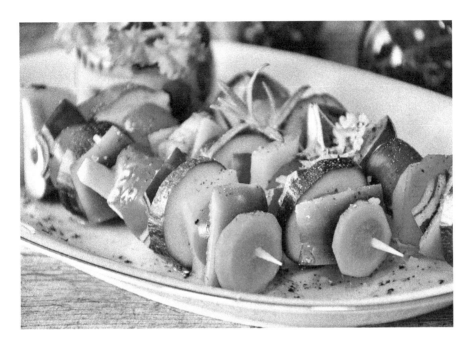

Hosting a party but not sure which appetizers to prepare as most of your guests are vegetarians? No worries as I have included some great vegetarian recipes for appetizers in this section.

Buffalo Cauliflower
Total Prep & Cooking Time: Thirty minutes

Yields: Twelve servings

Nutrition Facts: Calories: 120 | Protein: 4.2g | Carbs: 7.9g | Fat: 8.7g | Fiber: 2.3g

Ingredients:

- One serving of cooking spray
- Half cup of buffalo sauce

- Three tbsps. of mayonnaise
- One large egg
- Six cups of cauliflower florets
- Two cups of garlic croutons
- One-fourth cup of parmesan cheese (grated)

For the dipping sauce:

- One-fourth cup of each
  - Sour cream
  - Blue cheese salad dressing
- One tsp. of black pepper (ground)

Method:

1. Start by preheating your oven to 230 degrees Celsius. Use a cooking spray for greasing a baking tray.

2. Combine mayonnaise, buffalo sauce, and egg in a bowl. Toss the florets of cauliflower in the mixture of sauce and coat properly.

3. Spread the tossed florets on the baking tray.

4. Add the croutons on a blender and pulse them into crumbs. Add the cheese and pulse again. Spread the mixture of cheese and croutons over the florets of cauliflower.

5. Bake for fifteen minutes until tender and browned. Allow the florets to sit for five minutes.

6. Mix all the ingredients for the dipping sauce.

7. Serve cauliflower florets with dip sauce by the side.

Garlic Bread And Veggie Delight

Total Prep & Cooking Time: Thirty minutes

Yields: Five servings

Nutrition Facts: Calories: 390.2 | Protein: 12.4g | Carbs: 58.7g | Fat: 11.6g | Fiber: 7.2g

Ingredients:

- One cup of olive oil
- One garlic clove (chopped)
- One eggplant (cubed)
- One zucchini (cubed)
- One tomato (chopped)
- One tsp. of salt
- Two tsps. of each
  - Basil (minced)
  - Oregano (minced)
- One baguette
- Four tsps. of garlic powder
- Six tsps. of butter

Method:

1. Take a large skillet and add olive oil to it. Add garlic and fry for two minutes until browned.

2. Add the zucchini and eggplant to the skillet and cook for five minutes. Make sure that the eggplant is tender and brown.

3. Add the chunks of tomato and combine the veggies; add basil, oregano, and salt. Cook for two minutes and remove from heat.

4. Preheat oven 140/165 degrees Celsius.

5. Slice the baguette into one-inch slices, approximately twelve slices. Add butter and garlic powder on the bread slices and place them on the oven rack. Heat the bread for five minutes.

6. Arrange the heated bread slices on a plate. Top the slices with vegetables.

7. Serve immediately.

Spinach Parmesan Balls

Total Prep & Cooking Time: Thirty minutes

Yields: Ten servings

Nutrition Facts: Calories: 254.1 | Protein: 11.4g | Carbs: 18.4g | Fat: 14.2g | Fiber: 3.5g

Ingredients:

- Twenty ounces of frozen spinach (chopped)
- Two cups of bread crumbs
- One cup of parmesan cheese (grated)
- Half cup of butter (melted)
- Four green onions (chopped)
- Four eggs (beaten)
- Pepper and salt (for seasoning)

Method:

1. Start by preheating your oven at 175 degrees Celsius.

2. Take a bowl and combine spinach, bread crumbs, cheese, green onions, butter, pepper, salt, and eggs. Make balls of one-inch size from the prepared mixture.

3. Arrange the spinach balls on a baking tray. Bake for fifteen minutes until browned.

4. Serve hot.

Cheese Garlic Bread

Total Prep & Cooking Time: Thirty minutes

Yields: Eight servings

Nutrition Facts: Calories: 260 | Protein: 7.1g | Carbs: 29.7g | Fat: 11.4g | Fiber: 1.5g

Ingredients:

- Half cup of butter (melted)
- One tsp. of garlic salt
- One-fourth tsp. of rosemary (dried)
- One-eighth tsp. of each
    - Basil (dried)
    - Thyme (dried)
    - Garlic powder
- One tbsp. of parmesan cheese (grated)
- One loaf of French bread (halved)

Method:

1. Preheat oven at 150 degrees Celsius.

2. Mix garlic salt, butter, basil, rosemary, thyme, garlic powder, and cheese in a bowl.

3. Spread the butter mixture on the halves of the bread. Add extra cheese from the top if you want to.

4. Place halves of bread on a baking tray. Bake for twelve minutes until browned.

Stuffed Mushrooms

Total Prep & Cooking Time: Forty-five minutes

Yields: Twelve servings

Nutrition Facts: Calories: 89 | Protein: 2.6g | Carbs: 1.3g | Fat: 8.9g | Fiber: 0.6g

Ingredients:

- Twelve whole mushrooms
- One tbsp. of each
  - Minced garlic
  - Vegetable oil
- Eight ounces of cream cheese (softened)
- One-fourth cup of parmesan cheese (grated)
- One-fourth tsp. of each
  - Onion powder
  - Black pepper (ground)
  - Cayenne powder (ground)

Method:

1. Preheat the oven to 175 degrees Celsius. Grease a baking tray with the help of cooking spray.

2. Clean the mushrooms using a damp kitchen towel; break the stems. Chop the mushroom stems finely.

3. Take a skillet and heat oil in it. Add chopped stems of mushroom and garlic—Cook for five minutes.

4. Remove the skillet from heat and let it cool. Add the cream cheese, black pepper, parmesan cheese, cayenne powder, and onion powder. Mix well.

5. Use a small spoon for filling the mushroom caps with the mushroom stuffing.

6. Place the mushroom caps on the prepared baking tray.

7. Bake for twenty minutes until liquid forms under the mushroom caps.

Tomato Bruschetta

Total Prep & Cooking Time: Thirty-five minutes

Yields: Twelve servings

Nutrition Facts: Calories: 214.1 | Protein: 10.6g | Carbs: 23.1g | Fat: 8.8g | Fiber: 2.6g

Ingredients:

- Six tomatoes (chopped)
- Half cup of sun-dried tomatoes
- Three garlic cloves (minced)
- One-fourth cup of olive oil

- Two tbsps. of balsamic vinegar
- One-third cup of basil
- One-fourth tsp. of each
  - Black pepper (ground)
  - Salt
- One baguette
- Two cups of mozzarella cheese (shredded)

Method:

1. Preheat your oven on the setting of broiler.

2. Combine tomatoes, olive oil, vinegar, garlic, sun-dried tomatoes, basil, pepper, and salt in a bowl. Let the mixture sit for ten minutes.

3. Cut the baguette into slices of a three-fourth inch. Arrange the baguette slices on a baking tray. Broil for two minutes until browned.

4. Add the mixture of tomatoes on the slices of bread and top with mozzarella cheese.

5. Broil again for five minutes.

Spicy Pumpkin Seeds

Total Prep & Cooking Time: One hour and ten minutes

Yields: Eight servings

Nutrition Facts: Calories: 91 | Protein: 3.2g | Carbs: 8.8g | Fat: 4.9g | Fiber: 0.7g

Ingredients:

- Two tbsps. of margarine
- Half tsp. of salt
- One-eighth tsp. of garlic salt
- Two tsps. of Worcestershire sauce
- Two cups of pumpkin seeds (raw)

Method:

1. Preheat your oven at 135 degrees Celsius.

2. Combine the ingredients in a mixing bowl.

3. Bake for one hour. Stir in between.

Chapter 3: Soups & Side Dishes Recipes

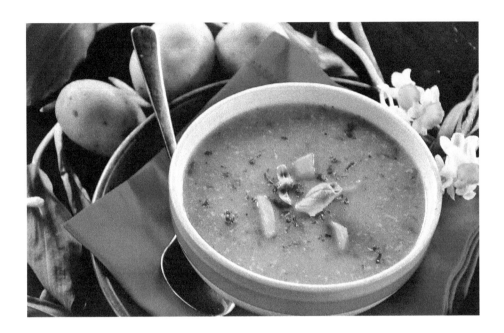

Soup forms an integral part of a vegetarian diet along with the side dishes. Here are some easy vegetarian recipes for side dishes and soups that you can include in your diet.

Carrot Soup
Total Prep & Cooking Time: Forty-five minutes

Yields: Four servings

Nutrition Facts: Calories: 351 | Protein: 3.2g | Carbs: 23.1g | Fat: 29.7g | Fiber: 4.2g

Ingredients:

- Two tbsps. of olive oil
- Four-hundred grams of carrots (cut in disks of half-inch)
- Half onion (diced)
- Four cloves of garlic (smashed)
- Two tsps. of cumin seeds
- Four cups of vegetable stock
- Two bay leaves
- One tsp. of salt
- One-fourth tsp. of white pepper
- Two tsps. of honey
- One-fourth cup of yogurt

Method:

1. Take a heavy bottom pan and add oil in it. Add onions, garlic, and cumin to the pan. Sauté on a medium flame for six minutes until tender and golden in color. Stir occasionally.

2. Add the stock, carrots, salt, bay leaves, white pepper, and simmer the mixture. Cover the pan and simmer for twenty minutes. Allow the soup to cool down for five minutes.

3. Use an immersion blender for blending the soup. Blend until you reach a silky smooth consistency.

4. Return the soup to heat and add honey. Stir the soup. Add yogurt and simmer. Taste the soup and adjust the seasonings. Keep the soup warm on very low flame until you serve.

5. Divide the soup among serving bowls. Serve with a dollop of yogurt from the top.

Note: You can use ground spices in place of the whole spices. But, whole spices will help in adding extra flavor.

Celery Soup

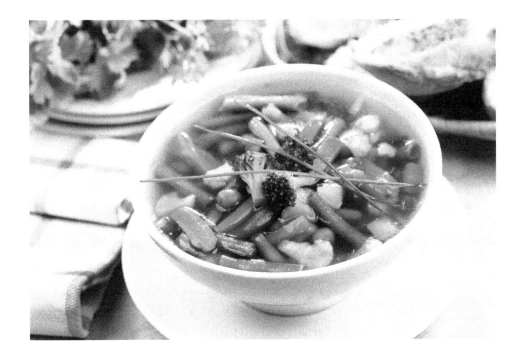

Total Prep & Cooking Time: Thirty-five minutes

Yields: Seven servings

Nutrition Facts: Calories: 180 | Protein: 4.2g | Carbs: 23.1g | Fat: 9.2g | Fiber: 4.9g

Ingredients:

- Two tbsps. of olive oil
- One onion (diced)
- Four cloves of garlic (chopped)
- Six cups of celery (thinly sliced)
- Two cups of potatoes (sliced in rounds)

- Four cups of vegetable stock
- One cup of water
- One bay leaf
- One tsp. of salt
- Half tsp. of pepper
- One-third tsp. of cayenne
- Half cup of sour cream
- One-fourth cup of each
  - Parsley (small stems)
  - Dill (small stems)

Method:

1. Take a large pot and add oil in it. Heat the oil and start adding the onion. Cook for five minutes until golden.

2. Roughly chop celery, potatoes, and garlic. Add garlic and cook the mixture for two minutes. Add potatoes, celery, stock, bay leaf, water, salt, cayenne, and pepper. The liquid needs to be enough to cover the vegetables. Cover the pot and boil the mixture. Simmer for ten minutes.

3. Remove bay leaf after turning off the stove. Add herbs to the pot and allow them to wilt.

4. Take an immersion blender and start blending the soup until silky smooth.

5. Return the pot to heat and cook over low flame for five minutes.

6. Serve with sour cream from the top.

Tomato Soup And Halloumi Croutons

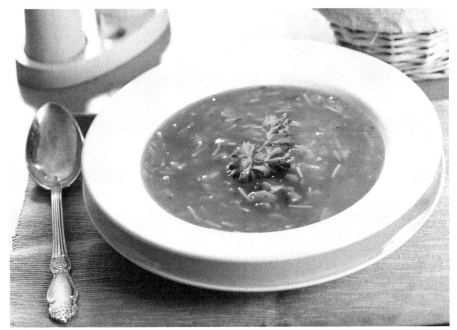

Total Prep & Cooking Time: One hour and five minutes

Yields: Six servings

Nutrition Facts: Calories: 285 | Protein: 10.3g | Carbs: 13.2g | Fat: 23.2g | Fiber: 4.9g

Ingredients:

- Three pounds of tomatoes
- Half red onion (sliced in thin rings)
- Six cloves of garlic
- Two tsps. of thyme leaves

- One-third cup of oil
- Four cups of vegetable stock
- One-fourth cup of basil leaves (chopped)
- One cup of Greek yogurt

For croutons:

- One block of halloumi cheese (cut in cubes of three-fourth inch)
- One tbsp. of oil

Method:

1. Start by preheating your oven at 200 degrees Celsius.

2. Use parchment paper for lining baking sheet. Spread the onions, tomatoes, and garlic on the sheet. Drizzle with some oil from the top—roast in the oven for thirty minutes.

3. Heat some oil in a pan and start adding the halloumi cubes. Cook for four minutes until golden on all sides.

4. Add the roasted veggies in a pot along with the vegetable stock. Use an immersion blender for blending the soup until smooth. Place the pot over a low flame and add seasonings of your choice. Simmer the soup and add basil. Simmer for ten minutes.

5. Add half a cup of yogurt to the soup.

6. Serve the soup in serving bowls with croutons from the top.

Baked Potatoes And Mushrooms With Spinach

Total Prep & Cooking Time: Forty-five minutes

Yields: Four servings

Nutrition Facts: Calories: 235.1 | Protein: 7.1g | Carbs: 27.1g | Fat: 11.3g | Fiber: 4.9g

Ingredients:

- One pound of potatoes (halved)
- Three tbsps. of olive oil
- Half pound of Portobello mushroom
- Six garlic cloves
- Two tbsps. of thyme (chopped)
- One pinch of black pepper and salt
- One-fourth cup of cherry tomatoes
- Half cup of spinach (sliced)
- Two tbsps. of pine nuts (toasted)

Method:

1. Preheat your oven at 200/220 degrees Celsius.

2. Add the potatoes in a roasting pan and drizzle some oil from the top. Roast the potatoes for fifteen minutes.

3. Add mushrooms along with garlic to the pan. Add thyme from the top along with some olive oil. Sprinkle black pepper and salt. Roast again for five minutes.

4. Add cherry tomatoes to the pan. Cook again for five minutes until the mushrooms are tender.

5. Add toasted pine nuts from the top and serve with spinach by the side.

Garlic Potatoes

Total Prep & Cooking Time: Fifty minutes

Yields: Four servings

Nutrition Facts: Calories: 270.2 | Protein: 5.2g | Carbs: 39.7g | Fat: 12.1g | Fiber: 4.9g

Ingredients:

- Two pounds of red potatoes (quartered)
- One-fourth cup of butter (melted)
- Two tsps. of garlic (minced)
- One tsp. of salt
- One lemon (juiced)
- One tbsp. of parmesan cheese (grated)

Method:

1. Start by preheating the oven at 175 degrees Celsius.

2. Place the potatoes in a baking dish.

3. Combine butter, lemon juice, garlic, and salt in a small bowl. Add this mixture over the potatoes and stir for coating. Add parmesan cheese from the top.

4. Bake the potatoes by covering the dish in the preheated oven for thirty minutes. Remove the cover and bake again for ten minutes.

Buttery Carrots

Total Prep & Cooking Time: Twenty-five minutes

Yields: Four servings

Nutrition Facts: Calories: 182.3 | Protein: 0.8g | Carbs: 21.3g | Fat: 10.3g | Fiber: 3.9g

Ingredients:

- One pound of baby carrots
- One-fourth cup of margarine
- One-third cup of brown sugar

Method:

1. Cook the baby carrots in boiling water. Drain most of the liquid leaving behind a little bit of liquid at the base.

2. Remove the carrots from the pot. Add brown sugar along with margarine. Simmer the mixture for two minutes and add the carrots to the pot. Toss well for combining.

3. Serve warm.

Chapter 4: Main Course Recipes

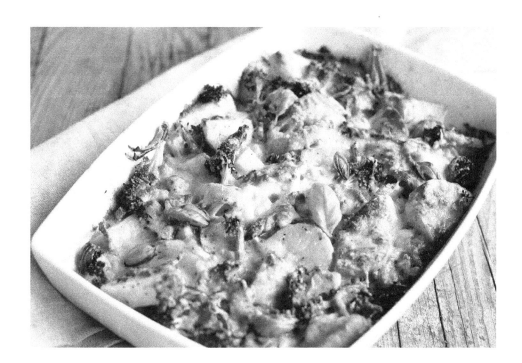

After you are done with the soups and side dishes, now it is time to jump into the main course. Here are some tasty main course recipes that you can include within your vegetarian diet plan.

Nut And Tofu Loaf

Total Prep & Cooking Time: One hour and forty minutes

Yields: Six servings

Nutrition Facts: Calories: 308.3 | Protein: 15.2g | Carbs: 27.6g | Fat: 14.2g | Fiber: 4.8g

Ingredients:

- One serving of cooking spray
- Twelve ounces of tofu (firm, drained, cubed)
- Two large eggs
- One ounce dry mix of onion soup
- One tbsp. of soy sauce
- Three-fourth cup of walnuts (chopped)
- One tsp. of olive oil
- Eight ounces of fresh mushrooms (sliced)
- One onion (chopped)
- Two celery stalks (chopped)
- Two tsps. of oregano (dried)
- One and a half tsps. of basil (dried)
- Half tsp. of sage (dried)
- Two cups of bread crumbs

Method:

1. Start by preheating the oven at 175 degrees Celsius. Use a cooking spray for greasing loaf pan.

2. Place eggs, tofu, soy sauce, and onion soup mix in a blender. Blend the ingredients until properly combined. Add the walnuts and blend again. Transfer the mixture of tofu to a bowl.

3. Take a large skillet and heat oil in it. Add mushrooms and cook them for four minutes. Add celery and cook for two minutes—season with basil, sage, and oregano.

4. Stir bread crumbs and veggies into the mixture of tofu. Press the loaf mixture into the pan.

5. Bake the loaf in the oven for sixty to seventy minutes.

6. Let the loaf cool down for five minutes before serving.

7. Slice the loaf and serve warm.

Velvety Chickpea Curry

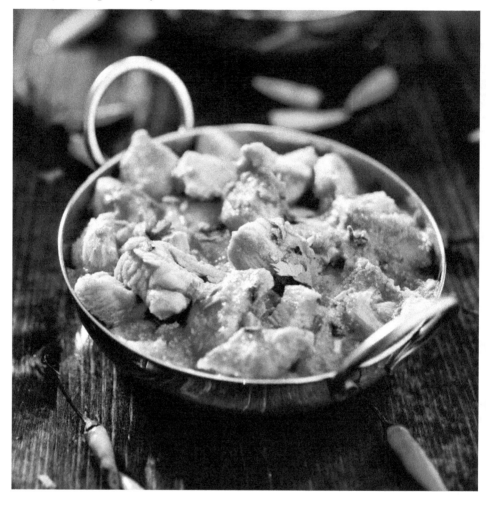

Total Prep & Cooking Time: Forty-five minutes

Yields: Six servings

Nutrition Facts: Calories: 408.3 | Protein: 10.2g | Carbs: 68.3g | Fat: 11.2g | Fiber: 8.9g

Ingredients:

- One tbsp. of each
  - Ginger root (minced)
  - Coconut oil
- One onion (sliced)
- Four garlic cloves (minced)
- Two tbsps. of curry powder
- One-fourth tsp. of pepper flakes
- Three cups of vegetable stock
- Two tbsps. of each
  - Soy sauce
  - Tomato paste
  - Maple syrup
- Half pound of potatoes (cut in pieces of a three-fourth inch)
- One carrot (sliced)
- Four cups of cauliflower florets
- One can of chickpeas (rinsed)
- Half cup of coconut milk
- One-fourth cup of cilantro (chopped)
- Half cup of peas (frozen)
- Salt (for seasoning)

Method:

1. Take a heavy-based pot and melt coconut oil in it. Add onions to the pot and sauté for five minutes. Add garlic and ginger to the pot—Cook for thirty seconds. Add pepper flakes, curry powder, soy sauce, stock, tomato paste, and maple syrup. Stir well.

2. Add carrots and potatoes to the pot and cover. Boil the mixture. Slightly open the cover and simmer for ten minutes. Add chickpeas, cauliflower, cilantro, and coconut milk. Stir well for combining. Simmer again for seven minutes. Add peas and cook for one minute.

3. Season with salt and cook for one minute.

4. Serve with basmati rice and cilantro from the top.

Tofu Pad Thai

Total Prep & Cooking Time: Forty-five minutes

Yields: Four servings

Nutrition Facts: Calories: 451 | Protein: 15.4g | Carbs: 60.1g | Fat: 15.2g | Fiber: 4.2g

Ingredients:

- Twelve ounces of tofu (drained, cubed)
- One tbsp. of cornstarch
- Three tbsps. of vegetable oil
- Eight ounces of rice noodles

For the sauce:

- One-fourth cup of each
  - Sriracha sauce
  - Water
  - Soy sauce
- Two tbsps. of white sugar
- One tbsp. of tamarind concentrate
- One tsp. of pepper flakes
- One large egg
- Two tbsps. of spring onions (chopped)
- One and a half tbsp. of peanuts (crushed)

- One lime (cut in wedges)

Method:

1. Coat the tofu cubes with cornstarch in a large bowl.

2. Heat two tbsps. of oil in a skillet. Fry the coated tofu for two minutes on each side.

3. Place the rice noodles in a medium bowl. Cover the noodles using hot boiling water. Soak the noodles until soft for three minutes. Drain the water.

4. Mix sriracha sauce, water, sugar, soy sauce, pepper flakes, and tamarind concentrate in a skillet. Cook for five minutes.

5. Heat one tbsp. of oil in a large wok. Add noodles, onion, along with the tofu. Cook the mixture for three minutes. Add sauce and toss it for combining.

6. Push the noodles to a side and crack the egg in the center. Stir for thirty seconds and mix with the noodles.

7. Serve with peanuts, green onion, and wedges of lime.

Eggplant Parmesan

Total Prep & Cooking Time: One hour

Yields: Ten servings

Nutrition Facts: Calories: 480.2 | Protein: 21.2g | Carbs: 60.1g | Fat: 15.2g | Fiber: 9.8g

Ingredients:

- Three eggplants (sliced)
- Two eggs (beaten)
- Four cups of bread crumbs
- Six cups of spaghetti sauce
- Sixteen ounces of mozzarella cheese (shredded)
- Half cup of parmesan cheese
- Half tsp. of basil (dried)

Method:

1. Preheat the oven at 175 degrees Celsius.

2. Dip the slices of eggplant in egg and then coat in bread crumbs.

3. Arrange the slices of eggplant in a baking sheet and bake for five minutes on both sides.

4. Take a baking dish and spread the spaghetti sauce for covering the base. Arrange the eggplant slices over the sauce. Sprinkle cheese from the top. Repeat for the remaining layers. Top with basil and cheese.

5. Bake for thirty-minutes until browned.

Veg Korma

Total Prep & Cooking Time: Fifty-five minutes

Yields: Four servings

Nutrition Facts: Calories: 451 | Protein: 8.4g | Carbs: 40.1g | Fat: 30.2g | Fiber: 8.7g

Ingredients:

- Two tbsps. of vegetable oil
- One onion (diced)
- One tsp. of ginger root (minced)
- Four garlic cloves (minced)
- Two potatoes (cubed)
- Four carrots (cubed)
- One jalapeno pepper (sliced)
- Three tbsps. of cashews (ground)
- One can of tomato sauce
- Two tsps. of salt
- One and a half tbsps. of curry powder
- One cup of green peas (frozen)
- One red bell pepper (roughly chopped)
- One-third yellow bell pepper (roughly chopped)
- One bunch of cilantro
- Half cup of heavy cream

Method:

1. Take a skillet and heat oil in it. Add onions to the oil and cook until soft. Add garlic and ginger to the skillet. Cook for one minute. Add carrots, potatoes, cashews, jalapenos, and tomato sauce. Add curry powder and season with salt. Stir well and cook for ten minutes until the potatoes are soft.

2. Add bell pepper, peas, and cream. Lower the flame and cover the skillet—Cook for ten minutes.

3. Serve with cilantro from the top.

Mac And Cheese

Total Prep & Cooking Time: Fifty minutes

Yields: Six servings

Nutrition Facts: Calories: 456 | Protein: 24g | Carbs: 33.1g | Fat: 24.9g | Fiber: 2.3g

Ingredients:

- Two cups of elbow macaroni (uncooked)
- One-fourth cup of butter
- Two tbsps. of flour
- One tsp. of each
  - Black pepper (ground)
  - Mustard powder
- Two cups of milk
- Eight ounces of each
  - Cheese food (cubed)
  - American cheese (cubed)
- Half cup of bread crumbs

Method:

1. Preheat the oven at 180/200 degrees Celsius. Take a casserole dish and grease with butter.

2. Boil water in a pot with salt. Add the pasta and cook the pasta for six minutes. Drain the water.

3. Take a saucepan. Melt butter in it. Add mustard powder, flour, and pepper. Add milk and stir constantly. Add the cheeses and mix for two minutes until the sauce thickens.

4. Add the macaroni to the cheese mixture. Mix well.

5. Transfer the pasta mixture to the greased dish. Add bread crumbs from the top.

6. Bake for twenty minutes by covering the dish.

7. Serve hot.

Sesame Noodles

Total Prep & Cooking Time: Thirty minutes

Yields: Eight servings

Nutrition Facts: Calories: 365.2 | Protein: 7.3g | Carbs: 51.1g | Fat: 13.2g | Fiber: 3.9g

Ingredients:

- Sixteen ounces of linguine pasta
- Six garlic cloves (minced)
- Six tbsps. of each
  - Safflower oil
  - Sugar
  - Rice vinegar
  - Soy sauce
- Two tsps. of chili sauce
- Two tbsps. of sesame oil
- Six green onions (sliced)
- One tsp. of sesame seeds (toasted)

Method:

1. Boil water in a large pot along with some salt. Add the pasta. Keep cooking for eight minutes. Drain all the water.

2. Take a saucepan and heat oil in it. Add garlic, sugar, soy sauce, chili sauce, and sesame oil. Boil the mixture until the sugar gets dissolved.

3. Add the sauce to the cooked pasta and toss well for combining.

4. Serve with sesame seeds and green onions from the top.

Chapter 5: Dessert Recipes

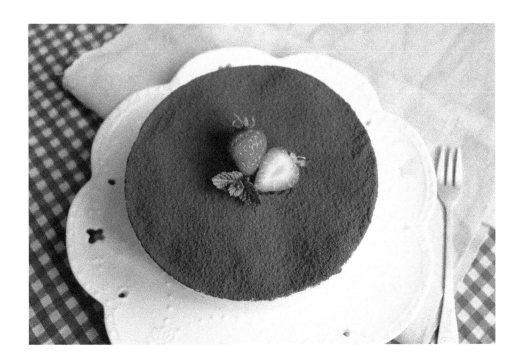

Having a great dessert after a tasty meal can make you, as well as your stomach, feel good. So, here are some vegetarian dessert recipes for you.

Raspberry And Rosewater Sponge Cake
Total Prep & Cooking Time: Fifty-five minutes

Yields: Ten servings

Nutrition Facts: Calories: 441 | Protein: 4.1g | Carbs: 51.3g | Fat: 23.1g | Fiber: 1.3g

Ingredients:

- Two-hundred grams of butter (softened)
- Two-hundred and fifty grams of caster sugar
- Four eggs (beaten)
- One tsp. of vanilla extract
- Two cups of flour

For the rose filling:

- Half cup of double cream
- One tsp. of rosewater
- Four tbsps. of raspberry jam
- One-third cup of raspberries (crushed)

For rose icing:

- Half cup of icing sugar
- Half tsp. of rosewater

Method:

1. Heat the oven at 160 degrees Celsius.

2. Use parchment paper for lining two baking tins—grease with butter.

3. Mix sugar and butter in a bowl. Add the eggs and mix again.

4. Add vanilla extract to the egg mixture and mix. Add flour and fold.

5. Divide the cake batter into the prepared baking tins and bake in the oven for twenty minutes. Let the cakes cool for ten minutes.

6. Whisk double cream along with rosewater. Add the jam and mix.

7. Place one of the cakes on a serving plate and add the cream mixture. Add raspberries from the top and place the other cake on top.

8. Mix all the ingredients for the icing.

9. Serve the cake with rose icing from the top.

Easy Tiramisu

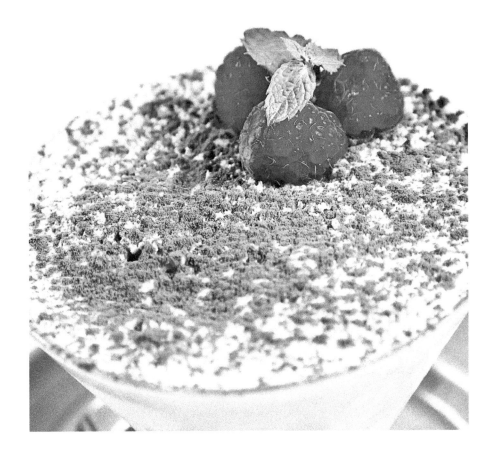

Total Prep & Cooking Time: One hour and fifteen minutes

Yields: Two servings

Nutrition Facts: Calories: 741 | Protein: 11.3g | Carbs: 44.3g | Fat: 51.6g | Fiber: 1.9g

Ingredients:

- Three tsps. of coffee granules
- Three tbsps. of coffee liqueur
- One and a half cup of mascarpone
- Half cup of condensed milk
- Six sponge fingers
- One tbsp. of cocoa powder

Method:

1. Mix coffee granules in two tbsps. of boiling water and stir for combining. Add three tbsps. of cold water along with coffee liqueur. Pour the mixture in a dish and keep aside.

2. Beat condensed milk, mascarpone, and vanilla extract in a bowl using a hand blender.

3. Break the fingers into two pieces and soak them in the mixture of coffee for thirty seconds.

4. Take a sundae glass and add the sponge fingers at the base. Add the cream mixture on top. Sift cocoa powder and chill in the refrigerator for one hour.

Chocolate Marquise

Total Prep & Cooking Time: Two hours and fifty-five minutes

Yields: Ten servings

Nutrition Facts: Calories: 710.3 | Protein: 7.8g | Carbs: 59.8g | Fat: 53g | Fiber: 1.5g

Ingredients:

- Three-hundred grams of dark chocolate
- Half cup of each
    - Caster sugar
    - Butter (softened)
- Six tbsps. of cocoa powder
- Six eggs
- One-third cup of double cream
- One-fourth cup of mint chocolate

Method:

1. Break the dark chocolate in small pieces and melt it using a double boiler system.

2. Beat butter and sugar in a bowl until creamy.

3. Separate the egg whites and yolks.

4. Mix the yolks with the sugar mixture until creamy.

5. Whip the double cream in another bowl.

6. Add the melted chocolate in the mixture of butter and fold gently. Add the whipped cream and mix well.

7. Spoon the mixture of chocolate in a piping bag.

8. Take a baking tin and pipe one layer of chocolate at the base of the tin. Cover the tin with pieces of mint chocolate. Repeat for the other layers. You will need to make four layers of mint chocolate.

9. Cover the tin with a cling film.

10. Chill the marquise in the fridge for two hours.

11. Remove the marquise from the tin by using a sharp knife.

12. Serve by cutting into slices.

Lemon Syllabub

Total Prep & Cooking Time: Fifteen minutes

Yields: Four servings

Nutrition Facts: Calories: 328 | Protein: 2.2g | Carbs: 14.6g | Fat: 28.6g | Fiber: 0.2g

Ingredients:

- Two cups of whipping cream
- Half cup of caster sugar
- Three tbsps. of white wine
- Half a lemon (juice and zest)
- Berries (for serving)

Method:

1. Mix sugar and whipping cream in a bowl. Whip until soft peaks are formed.

2. Add white wine in the mixture. Mix well. Add lemon juice and lemon zest in the mixture. Combine the ingredients properly.

3. Spoon the mixture into serving bowls or glasses.

4. Sprinkle remaining lemon zest from the top.

5. Serve the lemon syllabub with berries.

Note: You can use a mix of berries or only one type of berry.